Blueberry, Tomato & CoQ10 Antioxidants

(ANTHOCYANINS, LYCOPENE & UBIQUINONE)
CLAIMS VS. FACTS

BY
Prof Randolph M Howes MD,PhD
Physician, Surgeon and Scientist (Biochemist)

A CRITIQUE & REVIEW

Blueberry, Tomato & CoQ10 Antioxidants

(ANTHOCYANINS, LYCOPENE & UBIQUINONE)
CLAIMS VS. FACTS

BY
Prof Randolph M Howes MD,PhD
Physician, Surgeon and Scientist (Biochemist)

**Adjunct Assistant Professor of Plastic Surgery, (RET.)
The Johns Hopkins Hospital, Baltimore, MD USA**

**Espaldon Professor of Plastic and Reconstructive Surgery,
University of Santo Tomas, Manila, Philippines**

**Adjunct Professor of Biological Sciences,
Southeastern Louisiana University**

**Founder, Director and Chairman of the Scientific Advisory Board;
U.S. Medical Scientific Research Foundation, Inc.**

drug therapy are required. The author and the publisher of this work have checked with sources believed to be reliable in their efforts to provide information that is complete and generally in accord with the standards accepted at the time of publication. However, in view of the possibility of human error or changes in the medical sciences, neither the authors nor the publisher nor any other party who has been involved in the preparation of publication of this work warrants that the information contained herein is in every respect accurate or complete, and they disclaim all responsibility to any errors or omissions or for the results obtained from use of the information contained in the work. Readers should confirm the information contained herein with other sources. For example and in particular, readers are advised to check the product information sheets (or labels) included in the package of each drug they plan to administer to be certain that the information contained in this work is accurate and that changes have not been made in the recommended dose or in the contraindications for administration. This recommendation is of particular importance in connection with new or infrequently used drugs, additives or supplements.

Disclaimers: Please note: only your personal physician or other health professional you consult can best advise you on matters of your health based on your medical history, your family medical history, your medication history, and how information from any of these databases may apply to you. Neither Dr. Howes nor any party involved in creating, producing or delivering this web site shall be liable for any damages arising out of access to or use of this material or web site, or any errors or omissions in the content thereof.

The information given herein is not intended as medical advice. Always consult with your doctor for underlying illness. Before beginning dietary investigation, consult a dietician or a physician with an interest in nutrition. Information is drawn from the scientific literature, web research, and personal enquiry; while all care is taken, information is not warranted as accurate and the author cannot be held liable for any errors and omissions.

The information contained herein is not intended to replace a one-on-one relationship with a qualified health care professional and is not intended as medical advice. It is intended as a sharing of knowledge and information from the research of Dr. Howes. Dr. Howes encourages you to make your own health care decisions based upon your research and the advice of a qualified health care professional.

Financial disclosure: Dr. Howes has no financial conflicts of interest and is not involved in the sale of dietary supplements or fitness equipment. The author holds no stocks or interests in companies in the food additive or antioxidant supplement business.

ACKNOWLEDGEMENTS

Special thanks Don Neale Piatt, Sr. for proof reading.
Also, special thanks to Michael R. Root, M.S. for his unwavering encouragement.

The free radical theory
has more holes in it than
a warehouse full of Swiss cheese.
R. M. Howes, M.D., Ph.D.
1/2/15

I find the positive in everything,
even when there is none there.
My drive for accomplishment
and discovery
is only exceeded by my drive
to breathe.
R. M. Howes, M.D., Ph.D.
1/12/15

The story of antioxidants,
as they relate to disease
prevention, cure, and antiaging
is the story of ....
FAILURE!
R. M. Howes, M.D., Ph.D.
6/2/11

DEDICATION

**To CreateSpace, Amazon, and Jeff Bezos,
who have given me a world forum
for my ideas and efforts,
aimed at reducing the pain and suffering
of mankind.**

EMODs (electronically modified oxygen derivatives, previously called reactive oxygen species, ROS)
A mind constrained by misleading doggerel
is difficult to open
and impedes rational consideration
concerning emotional topics.
Ergo, it is necessary to distinguish fact
from manipulated myth,
to dispel generally accepted inaccuracies
and to challenge the power of the uninformed."
R. M. Howes, M.D., Ph.D.
3/4/04

"The cell's intracellular cytoplasmic sea is
an ocean of symphonic motion awash with
incomprehensible complexity."
R. M. Howes, M.D., Ph.D.
1/24/04

"The living/breathing cell is a cornucopia of
exciting electron affinities,
a thermodynamic treasure trove of biochemical
perplexities and
a temple of uncertainty for medical and scientific curiosity.

"With freshmanic amazement and sophomoric curiosity,
I study the hidden wonders and arcane secrets
of the aerobic cell.
What my peers see as a metabolic melee and free
radical fracas,
I view as a molecular marvel of unparalleled design.

Blueberry, Tomato & CoQ10 Antioxidants

(ANTHOCYANINS, LYCOPENE & UBIQUINONE)

CLAIMS VS. FACTS

TABLE OF CONTENTS:

SECTION ONE

BLUEBERRY ANTIOXIDANTS

(Anthocyanins)

INTRODUCTION

PROLOGUE

The meteoric rise of antioxidants and so-called "super foods" is a perfect example of how brilliant and aggressive marketing strategies can fool millions of uninformed consumers.

Some misguided notions are harmless but others are outright dangerous with deadly unintended consequences and can lead you down the road to chronic health problems, may even trim years off your life or result in your untimely and premature demise.

It is more important than ever, to distinguish fact from myth-information. In fact, it is becoming critical. Fortunately, the truth is slowly coming to the forefront as it relates to the free radi-crap theory and the harmful potential of ingesting excessive amounts of antioxidants.

Also surfacing is the essential protective and homeostatic role played by oxygen free radicals (i.e., electronically modified oxygen derivatives, EMODS; reactive oxygen species, ROS).

So-called dietary experts, public health authorities and nutritionists are frequently the least informed as to the dangers posed by excessive antioxidants. They cling to old, out dated, nullified theories and erroneous patterns of thinking.

Many antioxidant myths are perpetually repeated and begin to appear as truth. But, please do not be "radically misled" by this nonscience/nonsense.

The ridiculous notion that all EMODs are harmful arose from the invalidated free radical theory of the mid 1950s, as proposed primarily by the late Dr. Denham Harman. For half a century it dominated the thinking of scientists but has consistently fallen by the wayside of unproven hypotheses.

Investigators, such as myself, have combed the literature and I have offered over 500 studies showing the ineffectiveness of supplemental dietary antioxidants and have presented over 170 studies illustrating their harmful potential.

Still, marketing campaigns of persuasion have continued to hoodwink consumers and lead them astray with false claims referring to "miraculous cures, secret ancient remedies and super foods."

Truth in advertising is another giant myth, which only science based evidence can set straight.

Antioxidant after antioxidant has been exposed as being ineffective in prevention or the curing of a whole host of maladies. None have withstood rigorous scientific testing, especially with randomized controlled trials (RCTs). However, there are hints that a few may help with chronic eye diseases.

I have made my life's work the correction of the myths surrounding so-called antioxidants and to the enlightenment of oxidation/reduction chemistry (redox chemistry). Confusion is still rampant and misconceptions abound.

Super Doc discusses "super foods"

The misnomer "super foods" is tossed around with reckless abandon by today's marketers, when in actuality, there truly is no such thing. But, it sounds great.

Simply eat this super food and it will absolve you of all of you dietary indiscretions. At least, that is what they want you to believe.

However, today one can be a super Doc. On a number of occasions, I asked Bill Gates Sr. to express my deepest gratitude to his son, Bill Jr., for his contributions to the development of the internet.

I can literally sit in my study and with the click of a mouse, I can get more research done in a day than I could have done in a month in the Tulane Medical School library. All one has to have is the ability to assimilate massive amounts of data and the industriousness to work countless decades, and one can become a super Doc.

Today, I have benefits never before known to prior thinkers, such as Sir Isaac Newton, Ben Franklin and Albert Einstein.

I live in a blessed time.

I always aim to make it easier for the reader to understand the contents and message of my antioxidant books. Thus, I have included a summary section right in the front of the book, which is backed up by the studies subsequently presented. Actually, the repetition is good for the reader as a teaching device.

So, let's see what the blueberry, tomato and CoQ10 antioxidants hold in store for us. Are their claims hollow or are they factual?

Marketers continue to "sell" the public erroneous or exaggerated notions concerning the health benefits of antioxidants overall, but especially for blueberries.

The following are a few current titles which do exactly that:

Unleashing the Powers of Blueberries the Super Food!: Discover Exactly How To Release All The Remarkable Benefits. Aug. 12, 2013. By Marilyn Zeldon

Blueberries & Broccoli: A Scientist's Guide to Improving Your Odds with Cancer. Dec. 6, 2014. By Dr. George Ayoub.

Blueberries in Your Backyard: How to Grow America's Hottest Antioxidant Fruit for Food, Health, and Extra Money. Sept. 28, 2012. By R. J. Ruppenthal.

Now, let's start at the beginning.
In the following discussion, **the term "antioxidant" refers mainly to non-nutrient compounds in foods, such as polyphenols, which have antioxidant capacity** *in vitro* and so provide an artificial index of antioxidant strength – the ORAC measurement.
Other than for dietary antioxidant vitamins – vitamin A, vitamin C and vitamin E – no food compounds have been proved with antioxidant efficacy *in vivo*.

Accordingly, **regulatory agencies like the Food and Drug Administration (FDA) of the United States and the European Food Safety Authority (EFSA) have published guidance disallowing food product labels to claim an inferred antioxidant benefit when no such physiological evidence exists.** (FDA, 2008) (EFSA, 2010)

Summary of factoids on blueberry antioxidants

Things blueberries do not do:

- Studies have shown that berry anthocyanins are poorly bioavailable, are extensively conjugated in the intestines and liver, and are excreted in urine within 2–8 hours post consumption. (Kroon et al, 2004) (Netzel et al, 2002)

- The European Food Safety Authority (EFSA) is the body responsible for authorization of health claims within the European Union. The authorization of 222 out of 2758 health claims and their adoption by the European Commission on May 16 2012 has raised sound discussions within food industry. **None of the submitted berry claims have been authorized. So far, for none of the studied berries, including blueberries, is there a satisfactory (from the EFSA perspective) body of research available for substantiation of health claims related to antioxidant activities.** (Krasovskaya, 2012)

- The following blueberry-related claims have been withdrawn by the applicants:

- Claim nr. 3938: Vaccinium myrtillus (common name: blueberry, bilberry) – Astringent

- Claim nr. 2163: VitaBlue® Blueberry Extract 40% Total Phenolics – Excellent source of healthy fruit polyphenols known to help in the management of heart health

- Claim nr. 2162: VitaBlue® Wild Blueberry Extract – Excellent source of healthy fruit antioxidants. (EU register, 2012) **It could be concluded that available human trials were low-scale and operated with the markers which, if used alone, could not be considered**

sufficient for scientific substantiation of health claims from the EFSA's point of view. (Krasovskaya, 2012)

Research teams worldwide have no consensus as how to assess metabolism of (berry) flavonoids and their impact on health. Further (human) research is needed in order to design a reliable model for assessment of utilization of berries active compounds by the humans and their alleged benefits. (Krasovskaya, 2012)

It could be concluded that **available human trials were low-scale and operated with the markers which, if used alone, could not be considered sufficient for scientific substantiation of health claims from the EFSA's point of view.** (Krasovskaya, 2012)

As of 2012, the consumers should be aware that **sound claims of marketers on antioxidative properties of berries are not (sufficiently) substantiated from the scientific perspective.** As berries are a safe, tasty and nutrient-dense, their consumption should be encouraged. (Krasovskaya, 2012)

- Although the leaf extract has once been associated with a reduction in blood glucose, the fruits do not appear to inhibit carbohydrate absorption nor reduce fasting glucose.

- No known interactions with heart rate and blueberry supplementation.

- Blueberries do not appear to significantly influence nitric oxide metabolism.

- No significant influence on appetite or satiety.

- No known interactions with serum triglycerides following supplementation of blueberries.

- C-reactive protein does not appear to be influenced with blueberry supplementation.

- No significant changes in TNF-alpha concentrations.

- No significant influence on total cholesterol concentrations in the blood.

- No significant changes in LDL-C concentrations in serum with blueberries.

- No significant influence on HDL-C.

- Despite the reduction in muscle damage and increased rate of recovery, there are no significant changes in subjective muscle soreness.

- No significant influence on IL-6 concentrations in serum.

- Exercise-induced changes in cortisol are not influenced by blueberry supplementation.

- The study to measure nF-kB binding activity in muscle tissue after exercise failed to find an influence of blueberry supplementation.

- The lone study using a 2.5 hour running protocol at 72% VO2 max failed to find any significant differences between groups in oxidative status after exercise. Oral ingestion of 250g fresh berries daily for six weeks (and a single dose of 375g taken one hour before exercise) in well trained runners subject to 2.5 hours of moderate intensity exercise (72% VO_2 max) is able to **increase serum IL-10** relative to control and increase natural killer cell count by 76-122%, although **other immune cells (leukocytes, neutrophils, monocytes, and both T and B lymphocytes) and cytokines (IL-1ra, IL-6, IL-8) were unaffected**. (McAnulty et al, 2011)

- The alterations in most immune cells seen during exercise are wholly unaffected by blueberry supplementation. (McAnulty et al, 2011)

- Chronic loading of blueberries with an acute dose prior to prolonged exercise (2.5 hours) in trained men does not improve physical performance.

- Currently no studies noting changes in HbA1c, as it appears to be unaffected by supplementation.

- No significant influence on weight when taken as a daily supplement in obese individuals.

- No significant alterations in cell adhesion factors (sCAM-1 and vCAM-1).

- No significant influence on adiponectin concentrations in obese individuals.

(Human Effect Matrix For Blueberries, 2013) (http://examine.com/supplements/Blueberry/)

Other studies using rats and blueberries in the dosage range of 1-3% do not find significant alterations in food intake (appetite). (Yuji et al, 2013) (Clegg et al, 2011)

In **rats** fed blueberries or molecules after fermentation (phenylactic acid, hydroxylactic acid, and 3,4-dihydroxyphenylpropionic acid) **failed to reduce the hypertension caused by L-NAME**. (Xu et al, 2013)

Fresh blueberries (348mg anthocyanins) failed to influence blood flow, heart rate, or nitric oxide concentrations. (Del Bo et al, 2013)

Oral consumption of blueberry extract **daily for six weeks in obese and insulin resistant persons** failed to significantly alter HDL-C, LDL-C, or total cholesterol and these lipid biomarkers are unaffected with anthocyanins daily for eight weeks in persons at risk for cardiovascular disease. (Basu et al, 2010)

In guinea pigs fed a high cholesterol diet, blueberry ingestion failed to influence serum triglycerides (50% attenuation). (Coban et al, 2013)

Oral ingestion of fresh blueberries mixed into pancakes failed to significantly affect postprandial glucose absorption. (Clegg et al, 2011)

High dose anthocyanin has failed to reduce the postprandial spike in blood glucose, instead there was a slight increase 3-4 hours after ingestion. (Kay, Holub, 2002)

Blueberry fruits failed to reduce blood glucose in persons with insulin resistance or persons at risk for cardiovascular disease. A failure to benefit insulin sensitivity has been noted elsewhere in persons who were not insulin resistant. (Basu et al, 2010)

Blueberry polyphenols have failed to significantly increase lipolysis. (Moghe et al, 2012)

Weight gain and fat cell size as well as adipokines (leptin and adiponectin) are not affected by blueberry supplementation. (DeFuria et al, 2009)

Berries do not seem to be commonly consumed fruits by the US population, as documented in emerging nutrition and health research. (Bachman et al, 2008)

For blueberries, an age- and energy-adjusted model showed a significant decrease in coronary heart disease mortality, though the significance did not persist following adjustment for other confounding variables. For both strawberries and blueberries, the significant reduction in relative risk was associated with at least once per week consumption. A **mean anthocyanin intake of 0.2 mg/day was associated with a significantly reduced risk of CVD mortality in these postmenopausal women.** (Mink et al, 2007)

In contrast, blueberry intake was also examined in the Women's Health Study and no significant association was reported with risks of CVD or CRP. (Sesso et al, 2007)

None of these clinical studies showed any significant effect of berry intervention on biomarkers of inflammation, with the exception of a significant decrease in adhesion molecules following cranberry juice supplementation in healthy volunteers. (Ruel et al, 2008)

While it is alleged that antioxidants play a pivotal role in countering free radical activity within the body, **research investigating classical antioxidant supplementation (such as vitamin C and E) on the rate of recovery from exercise-induced muscle damage (EIMD), particularly functional recovery, has consistently shown little or no benefit from supplementation.** (Goldfarb et al, 2011) (McGinley, Shafat, 2009) (Nieman, Stear, 2010) (Wu et al, 2004)

Other reports either show that antioxidants have no action or have the ability to induce pro-oxidant effects. (Yfanti et al, 2010) (McAnulty et la, 2005) (Nieman et al, 2004)

Things blueberries are claimed to do:

- DNA damage appears to be acutely decreased following consumption of blueberries or its extracts (375mg anthocyanins or more) and tends to be in the range of a 20% reduction.

- Supplementation of blueberry extract does appear effective in elderly persons with general cognitive decline, able to improve cognition and memory.

- Memory formation in elderly subjects can be improved with daily supplementation of blueberries or their extract.

- Insulin has once been noted to be decreased in elderly persons with blueberry ingestion.

- A slight improvement in subjective well being and happiness has been noted in elderly persons given blueberries over a few weeks as a daily supplement.

- Oral ingestion of berries or their extracts tends to reduce oxidative biomarkers and improve antioxidant status either acutely or with daily supplementation.

- There appears to be a reduction in LDL oxidation, with the one chronic study suggesting a 27% reduction (the acute study noting less of a protective effect).

- A decrease in blood pressure has been noted in persons at risk for cardiovascular disease (6% systolic and 4% diastolic), but this may be limited to high risk individuals only.

- An improvement of insulin sensitivity has been noted in persons with insulin resistance, but this may only affect high risk individuals.

- Appears to reduce biomarkers of muscle damage such as creatine kinase.

- An increase in IL-10 following exercise has been noted.

- An increase in natural killer cells has been noted in the range of 76-122% following physical exercise.

- Alongside the reduction in serum oxidation comes a reduction in lipid peroxidation biomarkers such as MDA.

(Human Effect Matrix For Blueberries, 2013) (http://examine.com/supplements/Blueberry/)

Blueberry fruit are normally consumed as a whole fruit (fresh or frozen) and although they are low in vitamin C and E **they contain the**

broadest range of anthocyanin and polyphenolic antioxidant compounds among common berry fruits. (Wu et al, 2004)

Blueberry fruit exhibit a high antioxidant capacity (oxygen radical absorption capacity - ORAC) and have been shown to reduce oxidative stress and inflammation. (McAnulty et al, 2004) (Hurst et al, 2010)

In a study on cellular antioxidant activity of 25 common fruits wild blueberry was the champion in demonstrating antioxidant activity. Namely, wild blueberry had the highest phenolic content, the highest ORAC score and the highest cellular antioxidant activity. (Wolfe et al, 2008)

Blueberries also help maintain healthy blood flow via several mechanisms, including healthy low-density lipoprotein (LDL) oxidation, normal platelet aggregation, and maintenance of endothelial function. (Kalt et al, 2008) (Shaughnessy et al, 2009)

Blueberries are flowering plants of the genus *Vaccinium* with dark-purple berries, whose anthocyanins are considered to be nature's most potent antioxidants *in vitro*. (Srivastava et al, 2007)

Blueberries had the strongest total antioxidant capacity, and also had the highest TPC, TFC, and TAC, when compared to blackberries and strawberries.

The blueberries had particularly high levels of anthocyanidins and proanthocyanidins.

Blueberries are known to have a high anthocyanin content which confers relatively potent antioxidant potential *in vitro*, which has been noted to collectively confer about 85% of total antioxidant capacities of blueberries (the rest coming from other flavonoids). (Borges et al, 2010)

Exposure to high oxygen environments does not appear to negatively affect the anthocyanin content of blueberries, instead also causing a slight increase. (Zheng et al, 2003)

Blueberry-enriched diet ameliorates age-related declines in NMDA receptor-dependent long term potentiation (LTP). (Coultrap et al, 2008)

In cells exposed to TNF-α (proinflammatory molecule that can cause oxidation via NADPH oxidase activation from sphingolipids), 5µg/mL of blueberry extract can reduce oxidation to near control levels without affecting basal oxidation *in vitro.*

Blueberry polyphenols attenuate kainic acid-induced decrements in cognition and alter inflammatory gene expression in rat hippocampus. (Shukitt-Hale et al, 2008)

Similar benefits, to improve cognition in **aged rats** when fed in the diet at 0.004-0.016% over 12-13 weeks, **have been found with 2% blueberries in the diet, although this study attributed the observed benefit to anthocyanins**. (Andres-Lacueva et al, 2005)

In aged rats given 2% blueberries or the anthocyanin equivalent (179mcg/g), the improvements in spatial memory and attention performance were increased to an equal degree.

In twelve elderly humans with age-related memory decline, concord grape juice (6-9mL/kg, anthocyanin content not disclosed) daily for 12 weeks was **associated with an improvement of verbal learning with nonsignificant benefits in spatial and verbal recall** and a later study using similar dosing in a similar population found cognitive benefit with wild blueberry juice (428-598mg anthocyanins daily) as assessed by verbal memory tests. (Krikorian et al, 2010, BJNutr) (Kirkorian et al, 2010) **RMH Note: The small size of this study makes it questionable.**

A higher dietary intake of anthocyanins is associated with less risk for myocardial infarction in young and middle-aged women. (Cassidy et al, 2013) **RMH Note: There are studies showing no effect.**

Blueberries have been found to reduce blood pressure in hypertensive rats (spontaneously hypertensive rats) at 2-3% of the diet which has been replicated elsewhere. (Elks et al, 2011) (Shaughnessy et al, 2009)

In persons at risk for cardiovascular disease, freeze dried blueberries daily for eight weeks wa**s able to reduce both systolic (6%) and diastolic (4%) blood pressure.** (Basu et al, 2010)

Ingestion of 1% of the mouse diet as blueberries appears to be able to delay progression of atherosclerotic lesions in ApoE[-/-] **mice** without apparent changes in lipoprotein and triglyceride levels. (Wu et al, 2010)

Consumption of blueberries 10 and 5 hours before exercise is able to speed up the recovery of power following eccentric leg extensions, but does not appear to influence muscle soreness nor fatigue. (McLeay et al, 2012)

Antioxidant enzymes including SOD, Glutathione peroxidase, and catalase (reduced by DMBA toxin) have been noted to be preserved with blueberry (200mg/kg) and the reduction seen in hepatic fibrosis also abrogated. (Kavitha et al, 2013)

75µg/mL of blueberry anthocyanins or procyanidins have both been shown to reduce UV-induced DNA damage in cellular cultures. (Liu et al, 2013)

H_2O_2 induced DNA damage has been noted to be reduced in healthy controls (20% less oxidative damage). A single oral dose of blueberries was able to reduce H_2O_2 induced DNA damage from 51.7% to 42.7%. (Del Bo et al, 2013) However, the reduced DNA damage was very transient and disappeared after two hours and other studies using 200g of a mixed berry desert daily for two weeks have failed to find a significant change in basal DNA damage. (Carmen-Ramirez-Tortosa et al, 2004)

The phenolics of blueberries may possess anti-influenza properties *in vitro*. (Sekizawa et al, 2013)

The so-called oxidative stress induced by diethylnitrosamine is able to be attenuated with high dose blueberry supplementation in rats (5-10% of the diet) and blueberry juice has been noted to reduce fibrosis induced by CCL_4 over 8 weeks when consumed at 15g/kg daily. (Bingul et al, 2013) (Wang et al, 2013)

Supplementation of 2% blueberries in the diets of hypertensive rats is able to improve glomerular filtration rate and reduce renovascular resistance secondary to improving blood pressure. (Human Effect Matrix For Blueberries, 2013) (http://examine.com/supplements/Blueberry/)

Human intervention studies using chokeberries, cranberries, blueberries, and strawberries (either fresh, or as juice, or freeze-dried), or purified anthocyanin extracts have demonstrated significant improvements in LDL oxidation, lipid peroxidation, total plasma antioxidant capacity, dyslipidemia, and glucose metabolism. Benefits were seen in healthy subjects and in those with existing metabolic risk factors. (Basu et al, 2010)

Data reported from **the Kuopio Ischemic Heart Disease Risk Factor Study (KIHD) showed a significantly lower risk of CVD-related deaths among 1,950 men in the highest quartile of berry intake** (>408 g/day) versus men with the lowest intake (<133 g/day) during a mean follow-up of 12.8 years.

Analyses of NHANES data (1999–2002) revealed **a significant inverse association between serum CRP and anthocyanin intakes among US adults.** (Chun et al, 2008) Elevated CRP has been significantly associated with inflammation and is a high risk factor of CVD.

In an 8-week study, DeFuria et al. have shown **the attenuation of inflammatory gene expressions** in male C57Bl/6j mice fed a high-fat diet supplemented with blueberry powder versus the unsupplemented group. This study also showed **the protective effects of blueberries against insulin resistance and hyperglycemia, thus reducing the risk factors for CVD**. (DeFuria et al, 2009)

Purified anthocyanins from blueberries and strawberries prevented the development of dyslipidemia and obesity in mice fed a high-fat diet for a period of 90 days. (Prior et al, 2009)

Clinical studies in healthy humans, subjects with diabetes mellitus, dyslipidemia, metabolic syndrome, hypertension, or in smokers, show a significant decrease in CVD risk factors, especially glucose, lipids and lipid peroxidation, and systolic blood pressure, following berry intervention. (Basu et al, 2010)

RMH Note: As can be readily seen, there is lack of agreement of study results across the board, relative to blueberry consumption. One has to weigh the positive vs. the negative studies and arrive at their own conclusion.

Generally foods contain complex mixtures of polyphenols.

Polyphenols & Flavonoids

Blueberries also contain polyphenols and flavonoids. Consequently, I will include positive and negative studies on them from my book, *Chocolate, Red Wine Antioxidants (Polyphenols, Flavonoids & Resveratrol) Facts vs. Falsehoods.*

Summary of factoids on chocolate, red wine and resveratrol:

- More than 8,000 polyphenolic compounds have been identified in various plant species. (Kanti, Rizvi, 2009)

- Phenolic acids account for about one-third of the total dietary intake of polyphenols; flavonoids account for the bulk or the remaining two-thirds.

- Flavonoids can be further subdivided into 13 classes with more than 5,000 described compounds.

- Tea, wine, coffee, and cocoa contain hundreds of compounds other than polyphenols.

- In foods, all flavonoids except flavanols exist in glycosylated forms. (Kanti, Rizvi, 2009)

- The more processed chocolate is, the fewer flavonoids will remain.

- Milk products such as those found in milk chocolate can hinder the body's ability to efficiently absorb flavonoids and antioxidants from chocolate.

- The forms of polyphenols reaching the blood and tissues are different from those present in food and it is very difficult to identify all the metabolites and to evaluate their biological activity. (Setchell et al, 2003)

- Flavonoids vary widely in bioavailability, and most are poorly absorbed, undergo active efflux, and are extensively conjugated and metabolically transformed, all of which can affect the bioactive capacities (Harwood et al, 2007)

- Compared with the effects of polyphenols *in vitro,* **the effects** *in vivo,* **although the subject of ongoing research, are limited and vague.**

- Many purported health claims for specific polyphenol-enriched foods remain unproven.

- "Definitive conclusions on bioavailability of most polyphenols are difficult to obtain and further studies are necessary."

- One of the best studied, naturally occurring polyphenol stilbene is resveratrol (3,4',5-trihydroxystilbene), found largely in grapes.

- Flavonoids are poorly absorbed (usually less than 5%) and that what small amounts do get through to the circulation are rapidly metabolized to derivative compounds and excreted.

- In March 2007, scientists at the Linus Pauling Institute announced that flavonoids actually have little or no value as antioxidants and that their health benefits are likely the result of entirely different biochemical mechanisms.

- Dr. Frei discounts the antioxidant properties of flavonoids. In a media release, Dr. Balz Frei, professor of biochemistry and biophysics and director of the Linus Pauling Institute, was quoted as saying, "What we now know is that flavonoids are highly metabolized, which alters their chemical structure and diminishes their ability to function as an antioxidant.

- The large increase in total antioxidant capacity of blood observed after the consumption of flavonoid-rich foods is not caused by the flavonoids themselves, but is most likely the result of increased uric acid levels.

- A considerable amount of evidence is accumulating which supports the hypothesis that high-dose polyphenols can mechanistically cause adverse effects through prooxidative action.

- It has also been noted that plasma levels of conjugated flavonoids rarely, if at all, exceed 1 μmol/L. Clearly, absorption and ultimately bioavailability of polyphenols vary greatly and are complex.

- In red wine, up to 90% of the wine's phenolic content falls under the classification of flavonoids.

- In red grapes, the main flavonol is on average quercetin, followed by myricetin, kaempferol, laricitrin, isorhamnetin, and syringetin

- **Neither the FDA nor the EFSA has approved any health claim for flavonoids, or approved any flavonoids as pharmaceutical drugs.** (FDA, 2013)

- **Without any clinical studies, it is impossible to say if the antioxidant activity of grape-seed flavonoids offers any protection against oxidative stress in the human gastrointestinal tract**

- **There is no proof that chocolate is indeed an aphrodisiac.**

- **There is a popular belief that the consumption of chocolate can cause acne. This belief is not supported by scientific studies.**

Polyphenol Prooxidant Potential

- **Hot beverages contain high H2O2 concentrations because polyphenols oxidize rapidly at high temperatures.** Probably the most compelling supportive evidence involves studies of EGCG commonly found in tea. **H2O2 has been measured up to 19 umol/L in saliva of those chewing green tea leaves. EGCG undergoes, in vitro, oxidative polymerization and generation of H2O2 at concentrations up to 334 umol/L.** RMH Note: this illustrates their prooxidant potential.

- **Addition of catalase, an enzyme that specifically quenches H2O2, inhibits the death of human lung cancer cells incubated with EGCG.** In hepatocytes given high-dose EGCG (200 µmol/L), cell viability was significantly reduced and associated with increased ROS production and antioxidant, viz, glutathione, depletion.

RMH Note: This argues for prooxidant induced apoptosis and demonstrates the fact that antioxidants protect or shield cancer cells. RMH Note: the above indicates that polyphenols kill cancer cells oxidatively, not antioxidatively! This is the same pattern with most other compounds that have tumoricidal activity (i.e., EMOD-induced cancer apoptosis).

- **Hot beverages contain high H2O2 concentrations because polyphenols oxidize rapidly at high temperatures.** (Martin, Appel, 2010)

- H2O2 has been measured up to 19 umol/L in saliva of those chewing green tea leaves. EGCG undergoes, in vitro, oxidative polymerization and generation of H2O2 at concentrations up to 334 umol/L. (Martin, Appel, 2010)

- Addition of catalase, an enzyme that specifically quenches H2O2, inhibits the death of human lung cancer cells incubated with EGCG. (Martin, Appel, 2010)

- EGCG can undergo redox cycling and produce quinones with subsequent increases in oxidative stress (prooxidant activity). (Martin, Appel, 2010)

- Polyphenols can accept an electron to form relatively stable phenoxyl radicals, thereby disrupting chain oxidation reactions in cellular components. (Clifford, 2000)

- A considerable amount of evidence is accumulating which supports the hypothesis that high-dose polyphenols can mechanistically cause adverse effects through prooxidative action. (Martin, Appel, 2010)

Negative factoids (including toxicities)

- Antioxidants, including polyphenols, have been linked to numerous detrimental health conditions when taken in larger doses found in dietary supplements and fortified foods. (Martin, Appel, 2010)

- Some human intervention trials have shown not only failure to protect by polyphenols but accelerated development of cancers or CVD in susceptible subjects. (Halliwell, 2007)

- There have been a number of recent case reports of hepatotoxicity related to the consumption of high doses of polyphenol-enriched, tea-based dietary supplement (10-29 mg/kg/d).

- The theobromine found in chocolate is toxic to animals such as horses, dogs, parrots, small rodents, and cats

- Chocolate consumption may have potential to cause mild lead poisoning.

- **High-dose EGCG induced multi-organ toxicity associated with increased plasma levels beyond that normally encountered through diet**. (Martin, Appel, 2010)

- **Some human intervention trials have shown not only failure to protect by polyphenols but accelerated development of cancers or CVD** in susceptible subjects. (Halliwell, 2007)

- **There have been a number of recent case reports of hepatotoxicity related to the consumption of high doses of polyphenol-enriched, tea-based dietary supplement** (10-29 mg/kg/d). Concentrated preparations of polyphenol-rich green tea were dangerous and should be avoided. Several additional human case studies have shown hepatotoxicity related to the consumption of high-dose, tea-based dietary supplements. **All pathology resolved after the dietary supplement was discontinued although reinjury occurred with rechallenge.** (Martin, Appel, 2010)

- **Polyphenols can exhibit many adverse effects to diverse biological systems.** For example, **several flavonoids inhibit the enzyme thyroid peroxidase and interfere with thyroid hormone biosynthesis and ultimately thyroid function.** (Martin, Appel, 2010)

- **Elevated consumption of soy isoflavones can reduce fertility and retard sexual maturation.** (Martin, Appel, 2010)

- **Polyphenols can also exhibit anti-nutritional effects through complexation of minerals such as iron.** (Martin, Appel, 2010)

- **Larger molecular weight polyphenols, i.e., tannins, can interact with proteins and inhibit several enzymes that are needed for growth.** (Martin, Appel, 2010)

- **High polyphenol intake could also increase the risk of CVD through alterations in homocysteine processing, a well-accepted biomarker for CVD.** (Martin, Appel, 2010)

- **Polyphenols, specifically naringenin in grapefruit, can inhibit drug-metabolizing enzymes such as CYP3A4, among others, involved in xenobiotic metabolism and, thus, interact with pharmacological agents increasing the risk of overdose and harm.** (Kiani et al, 2007)

- **The transient ischemic attack-like symptoms could possibly be attributable to one or more components of the oolong tea.** (Layher et al, 2013)

- Many diverse polyphenols can affect the activities of many CYP450 enzymes other than 3A4 by induction and inhibition. (Martin, Appel, 2010)

- It seems especially dangerous to continue pushing excessive consumption of polyphenols in polyphenol-rich dietary products (fortified or enhanced food, food extract, or pure compound, i.e., dietary supplement), given their known harmful potential. (Martin, Appel, 2010)

- There was limited to moderate evidence that the consumption of green tea reduced the risk of lung cancer, especially in men, and urinary bladder cancer or that it could even increase the risk of the latter. (Boehm et al, 2009)

- Acute black tea consumption increased systolic blood pressure.

- A company called Sirtris Pharmaceuticals, which was established to develop drugs from resveratrol, pulled the plug on the program in 2010 when a clinical trial showed that one of these drugs might be linked to kidney damage. (Patrick J. Skerrett, Executive Editor, *Harvard Health*)

- In older men, a natural antioxidant compound found in red grapes and other plants -- called resveratrol -- blocks many of the cardiovascular benefits of exercise, specifically reduced blood pressure and cholesterol, according to research published today [22 July 2013] in *The Journal of Physiology*. (Gliemann et al, 2013)

- Research at the Linus Pauling Institute and the European Food Safety Authority shows that flavonoids are poorly absorbed in the human body (less than 5%), with most of what is absorbed being quickly metabolized and excreted. (EFSA, 2010)

- Clearly, absorption and ultimately bioavailability of polyphenols vary greatly and are complex. Bioavailability from dietary intake of polyphenols is 2%–20% so minimal amounts of dietary polyphenols are absorbed, with subsequently low levels found in plasma. (Martin, Appel, 2010)

- Circulating antioxidants such as glutathione, ascorbic acid, uric acid, tocopherols, and carotenoids are present in the body at concentrations thousands of times higher than the nanomolar plasma levels fleetingly achieved by polyphenols.

- **Flavonoids have negligible systemic antioxidant activity, and the increase in antioxidant capacity of blood seen after consumption of flavonoid-rich foods is not caused directly by flavonoids, but due to increased production of uric acid resulting from excretion of flavonoids from the body.** (Stauth, 2007)

- **The forms of ployphenols reaching the blood and tissues are different from those present in food and it is very difficult to identify all the metabolites and to evaluate their biological activity.** (Setchell et al, 2003)

- **Clinical studies investigating the relationship between flavonoid consumption and cancer prevention/development are conflicting for most types of cancer.** (Romagnolo, Selmin, 2012)

- **In test tubes, cocoa has antioxidant activity, an effect not proved in the body.**

- **Consuming milk chocolate or white chocolate, or drinking fat-containing milk with dark chocolate, appears to largely negate the health benefit.** (Serafini et al, 2003)

- **A follow-up study on the CARET study in the *Journal of the National Cancer Institute* in 2004 showed that the increased risk of lung cancer persisted for years after the beta-carotene and retinal supplementation had ceased.** (Goodman et al, 2004)

- It is clear that **the data are confusing and self-contradictory, regarding the in vivo role of polyphenolics.** (Wiseman et al, 2000)

- **Any effect on any measurable parameter observed with fruit juices, beverages, soy products, or vegetables is not necessarily an effect of the flavonoids or other phenolic compounds that the products contain.** (Halliwell et al, 2005)

- **The real contributions of such compounds to health maintenance and the mechanisms through which they act are still unclear.** (Halliwell et al, 2005)

- **The available literature provides no consistent support for systemic antioxidant effects of dietary phenolic compounds.** (Halliwell et al, 2005)

- **It must not be assumed that any protective effect of flavonoid-rich foods is attributable to antioxidant actions of the**

flavonoids or to flavonoids at all, rather than to other components in the foods. (Cao, Cao, 1999)

- Some studies suggest that flavonoid intake was not associated with reduced CHD. (Rimm et al, 1996)

- The mechanism underlying the effects of flavonoids/procy-
andins on the endothelium has yet to be defined (or proven).

- The medical literature is replete with reports of the beneficial properties of dietary polyphenols and also the possible adverse effects of
polyphenol-rich plants and their components as fortified, enhanced, or purified foods and/or dietary supplements. (Schilter
et al, 2003)

- Results from studies assessing associations between green
tea and risk of digestive tract cancer incidence were highly
contradictory. There was limited evidence that green tea
could reduce the incidence of liver cancer. The evidence for
esophageal, gastric, colon, rectum, and pancreatic cancer was
conflicting. (Boehm et al, 2009)

- There is insufficient and conflicting evidence to give any firm
recommendations regarding green tea consumption for cancer prevention. (Boehm et al, 2009)

- There is insufficient and conflicting evidence regarding flavonoid intake and the prevention of colorectal neoplasms. (Jin et al,
2012)

- There was no evidence that total flavonoid intake reduced
the risk of colorectal neoplasms. The evidence for Isoflavones,
Flavonols, Flavones and Flavanones was conflicting. (Jin et al,
2012)

- The biological relevance of direct antioxidant effects of polyphenols for cardiovascular health in humans is not established.
(Hollman et al, 2011)

- In the United Kingdom, tea was positively associated with
CHD. Tea consumption was positively associated with a less healthy
lifestyle and lower social class. (Hertog et al, 1997)

- An Italian case-control study and 2 cohort studies in Western
countries did not find an effect of isoflavones on CVD risk.

- Limited evidence is available to support an effect of red wine, chocolate, and green and black tea on triglyceride concentrations.

- Data from over 130 randomized clinical trials provide evidence for the effectiveness of some foods rich in flavonoids or polyphenols in reduction of CVD risk factors, but it is still not clear whether these beneficial effects can really be ascribed to the polyphenols contained in these foods or extracts. (Geleijnse, Hollman, 2008)

- There is limited evidence that polyphenol-rich products or polyphenols are able to decrease lipid peroxidation.

- Results from RCTs in human athletes with large doses of purified flavonoids such as quercetin have been disappointing. (Nieman, 2010)

- In 2012, the University of Connecticut announced that it had concluded that Dipak K. Das, Ph.D., a professor in its Department of Surgery and director of the Cardiovascular Research Center, was guilty of 145 counts of fabrication and falsification of (resveratrol) data and that the university had notified eleven journals about this problem. (UConn Today, 2012)

- Das had gained attention for his reports on allegedly beneficial properties of resveratrol. As of June 2012, four of the journals have retracted twelve of his papers, many of which were repeatedly cited by others. (Oransky, 2012)

- In 2011, a systematic review with 21 co-authors noted that people are consuming resveratrol concluded that, "the published evidence is not sufficiently strong to justify a recommendation for the administration of resveratrol to humans, beyond the dose which can be obtained from dietary sources." (Vang et al, 2011)

- Study into the cardioprotective effects of resveratrol is based on the research of Dipak K. Das. However, he has been found guilty of scientific fraud, and many of his publications related to resveratrol have been retracted. (Weir et al, 2012)

- On May 5, 2010, however, GlaxoSmithKline (GSK) said it had suspended a small clinical trial of SRT501, a proprietary form of resveratrol, due to safety concerns, and terminated the study on December 2, 2010. (Clinical Trial.gov)

- The hypothesis that resveratrol from wine could have higher bioavailability than resveratrol from a pill has been refuted by experimental data. (Goldberg et al, 2003)

- The trace amounts of resveratrol reached in the blood are insufficient to explain the French paradox. The beneficial effects of wine apparently could be explained by the effects of alcohol or the whole complex of substances wine contains. (Corder et al, 2006)

- Cocoa powder, baking chocolate and dark chocolate also have low levels of resveratrol in normal consumption quantities (0.35 to 1.85 mg/kg). (Hurst et al, 2008)

- Resveratrol has not been tested in clinical trials, and most clinical trials of other antioxidants have failed to demonstrate the benefits suggested by preliminary studies.

- The polyphenol resveratrol, a compound found in red wine, grapes, and dark chocolate, does not increase longevity or reduce the risk of heart disease or cancer. (May 12, 2014 in the *Journal of the American Medical Association: Internal Medicine*)

- Conclusions and Relevance: In older community-dwelling adults, total urinary resveratrol metabolite concentration was not associated with inflammatory markers, cardiovascular disease, or cancer or predictive of all-cause mortality. Resveratrol levels achieved with a Western diet did not have a substantial influence on health status and mortality risk of the population in this study. (Semba et al, 2014)

- Similarly, there was no association between resveratrol concentrations and cancer risk, nor was there any association with inflammatory markers such as C-reactive protein (CRP), tissue necrosis factor (TNF), interleukin-6, and interleukin-1ß. (Semba et al, 2014)

- Enjoy red wine in moderation, but it isn't going to help you live longer or protect them against heart disease and cancer. (Semba et al, 2014)

- These results led researchers to conclude that resveratrols in our food have no measurable impact on our health. (Semba et al, 2014)

- The American Heart Association (AHA) doesn't recommend antioxidant supplements for cardiovascular risk reduction.

- The research that resveratrol blocks many of the cardiovascular benefits of exercise, adds to the growing body of evidence questioning the positive effects of antioxidant supplementation in humans. (Gliemann et al, 2013)

- Resveratrol did not elicit metabolic improvements in healthy aged subjects; in fact, resveratrol even impaired the observed exercise training-induced improvements in markers of oxidative stress and inflammation in skeletal muscle. (Olesen et al, 2014)

- Resveratrol -- an antioxidant found in red wine, chocolate, and grapes --didn't correlate with longevity or lower risk of cancer or cardiovascular disease when dietary intake was directly measured in a prospective study. (Semba et al, 2014)

- "You would need to drink a hundred to a thousand glasses of red wine to equal the doses that improve health in mice," says Dr. Sinclair.

- if one relied on red wine alone to gain the lasting effects found in studies of mice and rats, it would require drinking more than 60 liters a day.

- While 70% of orally administered resveratrol is absorbed its oral bioavailability is approximately 0.5% due to extensive hepatic gluconuridation and sulfation. Only trace amounts (below 5 ng/ml) of unchanged resveratrol could be detected in the blood after 25 mg oral dose. (Walle et al, 2004)

- Various plant extract and agents such as resveratrol, catechins, EGCG, quercetin, gossypol, curcumin and caffeic acid have routinely been shown to induce damage to isolated plasmid DNA, albeit under certain conditions (e.g. in the presence of transition metal ions, especially copper). (Hadi et al, 2007)

- Recent clinical trials do not provide sufficient evidence for an essential contribution of cocoa products to the overall antioxidant defense. Any recommendations for cocoa intake within preventive and therapeutic measures are presently not reasonable. (Scheid et al, 2010)

- **This RCT investigation failed to support the predicted beneficial effects of short-term dark chocolate and cocoa consumption on any of the neuropsychological or cardiovascular health-related variables** included in this research. **Consumption of dark chocolate and cocoa was, however, associated with significantly higher pulse rates at 3- and 6-wk treatment assessments.** (Crews et al, 2008)

- **Our study did not find a blood pressure lowering effect of dark chocolate or tomato extract in a prehypertensive population.** (Reid et al, 2009)

- **Flavanol-rich chocolate did not significantly reduce mean blood pressure below 140 mmHg systolic or 80 mmHg diastolic.** (Reid et al, 2010)

Positive factoids

- **A cup of coffee contains around 100 mg polyphenols.** (Martin, Appel, 2010)

- **One of the best studied, naturally occurring polyphenol stilbene is resveratrol (3,4′,5-trihydroxystilbene), found largely in grapes.** (Kanti, Rizvi, 2009)

- **Some studies conducted in Europe, Asia, and North America have found that people who eat a diet rich in flavonoids from chocolate or cocoa have lower incidents of cancer than those who eat fewer flavonoids.** (Jacobi, 2008)

- **The American Heart Association (AHA) has stated that people who consume a bar-sized serving of flavonol-rich dark chocolate daily may lower their blood pressure and actually improve their blood sugar over the long run**

- **Men with the highest cocoa consumption were half as likely to die from cardiovascular disease.** (Ding et al, 2008)

- **High dietary consumption of flavanoids, specifically flavanols (or flavan-3-ols), through, for example, cocoa plant-based dark chocolate, is associated with reduced risk and prevalence of** cardiovascular disease and cardiovascular-related mortality. (Janszky et al, 2009)

- Dietary flavonoid intake is associated with reduced gastric carcinoma risk in women, and reduced aerodigestive tract cancer risk in smokers. (Gonzalez, et al, 2013)

- Long-term consumption of chocolate showed an increase of HDL cholesterol by 11% which appeared to be enhanced by addition of cocoa polyphenols. (Mursu et al, 2004)

- Clinical trials with dark chocolate, green tea, pomegranate, and Concord grape juice confirm benefits such as lower blood pressure, reduced platelet stickiness, and improved artery wall elasticity.

- Two other prospective trials suggested a lower risk of myocardial infarctions (MIs) with flavonoid intake. (Hirvonen et al, 2001)

- A total of eight cohort studies found lower congestive heart disease (CHD) mortality with total or specific flavonoid intake. (Hertog et al, 1995)

- Quercetin, a flavonoid prominent in onions and apples, has been epidemiologically linked with protection from coronary artery disease and cancer. (Ding et al, 2006) (Hirvonen et al, 2001)

- Chocolate derived from the plant *Theobroma cacao*, rich in flavonoids, have shown improved endothelium-dependent flow-mediated dilation (FMD). (Engler et al, 2004)

- Grapeseed extract has also been shown to be a more potent scavenger of oxygen-free radicals (an oxidative stressor) than other common antioxidants such as vitamin C and E. (Bagchi et al, 1997)

- Other potential benefits of grape seed extract (GSE) have been centered on its effect on neoplasia and there have been several encouraging trials undertaken suggesting a beneficial effect. (Moore, Morre, 2005)

- Long term consumption of diets rich in plant polyphenols offered some protection against development of cancers, cardiovascular diseases, diabetes, osteoporosis and neurodegenerative diseases. (Graf et al, 2005)

- **Epidemiological studies have repeatedly shown an inverse association between the risk of chronic human diseases and the consumption of polyphenolic rich diet.** (Scalbert et al, 2005) (Arts, Hollman, 2005) **RMH Note: Epidemiologic studies are the weakest and do not prove causality or anything else.**

- **A number of studies has demonstrated that consumption of polyphenols limits the incidence of coronary heart diseases.** (Renaud, de Lorgeril, 1992) (Dubick, Omaye, 2001) (Nardini et al, 2007)

- **Consumption of polyphenol rich diet have been associated with a lower risk of myocardial infarction in both case-control and cohort studies.** (Peters et al, 2001)

- **Effect of polyphenols on human cancer cell lines, is most often protective and induce a reduction of the number of tumors or of their growth.** (Yang et al, 2001)

- **The anti-carcinogenic effects of resveratrol appears to be closely associated with its antioxidant activity.** (Athar et al, 2007)

- **Numerous studies report the antidiabetic effects of polyphenols. Tea catechins have been investigated for their anti-diabetic potential.** (Rizvi et al, 2005) (Rizvi, Zaid, 2001)

- **People drinking three to four glasses of wine per day had 80% decreased incidence of dementia and Alzheimer's disease compared to those who drank less or did not drink at all.** (Scarmeas et al, 2007)

- **Administration of polyphenols provide protective effects against Parkinson's disease,** a neurological disorder characterized by degeneration of dopaminergic neurons in the *substantia nigra zona compacta.* (Aquilano et al, 2008)

- **A statistically significant reduced risk of colorectal cancer (CRC) was found with high intake of epicatechin.** (Jin et al, 2012)

- **Consumption of 3 or more cups of tea (green or black) per day lowered the risk of stroke by 21%.** (Arab, Elsahoff, 2009)

- **Among high-risk subjects, those who reported a high polyphenol intake, especially of stilbenes and lignans, showed a**

reduced risk of overall mortality compared to those with lower intakes. (Tresserra-Rimbau et al, 2014)

- The anticancer property of resveratrol has been supported by its ability to inhibit proliferation of a wide variety of human tumor cells in vitro. (Bishayee, 2009)

Natural phenols are a class of molecules found in abundance in plants.

More than 10,000 phytochemicals have been identified.

Several thousand polyphenols have been identified.

Approximately 8,000 individual flavonoids have been identified.

Approximately 400 individual anthocyanins (ACNs) have been identified.

Uric acid, in humans, accounts for roughly half the antioxidant capacity of plasma.

Fructose, which is found abundantly in fruits, significantly elevates uric acid levels in humans, and thus indirectly increases antioxidant capacity. (Zawiasa et al, 2009)

RMH Note: I believe that our current high fructose diets increase uric acid levels, which increase our antioxidant capacity and thus, decrease our prooxidant levels and create an EMOD insufficiency.

I believe this is the basis of today's high levels of cancer, heart disease, strokes, diabetes, arthritis, etc.

Although **some believe that high levels of uric acid may be a protective factor against Parkinson's disease and possibly other diseases related to so-called oxidative stress.** (De Vera et al, 2008)

Flavonoids

Flavonoids, a subset of polyphenol antioxidants, are present in many berries, as well as in coffee and tea.

- Flavones: Apigenin, Luteolin, Tangeritin
- Flavonols: Isorhamnetin, Kaempferol, Myricetin - walnuts are a rich source, Proanthocyanidins, or condensed tannins, Quercetin and related, such as rutin
- Flavanones: Eriodictyol, Hesperetin (metabolizes to hesperidin), Naringenin (metabolized from naringin)
- Flavanols and their polymers: Catechin, gallocatechin and their corresponding gallate esters, Epicatechin, epigallocatechin and their corresponding gallate esters, Theaflavin its gallate esters, Thearubigins
- Isoflavone phytoestrogens - found primarily in soy, peanuts, and other members of the Fabaceae family, Daidzein, Genistein, Glycitein
- Stilbenoids: Resveratrol - found in the skins of dark-colored grapes, and concentrated in red wine. Pterostilbene - methoxylated analogue of resveratrol, abundant in *Vaccinium* berries
- Anthocyanins: Cyanidin, Delphinidin, Malvidin, Pelargonidin, Peonidin, Petunidin

Phenolic acids and their esters

Main article: polyphenol antioxidants

- Chicoric acid - another caffeic acid derivative, is found only in the popular medicinal herb Echinacea purpurea.
- Chlorogenic acid - found in high concentration in coffee (more concentrated in robusta than arabica beans), blueberries and tomatoes. Produced from esterification of caffeic acid.
- Cinnamic acid and its derivatives, such as ferulic acid - found in seeds of plants such as in brown rice, whole wheat and oats, as well as in coffee, apple, artichoke, peanut, orange and pineapple.
- Ellagic acid - found in high concentration in raspberry and strawberry, and in ester form in red wine tannins.
- Ellagitannins - hydrolyzable tannin polymer formed when ellagic acid, a polyphenol monomer, esterifies and binds with the hydroxyl group of a polyol carbohydrate such as glucose.

- Gallic acid - found in gallnuts, sumac, witch hazel, tea leaves, oak bark, and many other plants.
- Gallotannins - hydrolyzable tannin polymer formed when gallic acid, a polyphenol monomer, esterifies and binds with the hydroxyl group of a polyol carbohydrate such as glucose.
- Rosmarinic acid - found in high concentration in rosemary, oregano, lemon balm, sage, and marjoram.
- Salicylic acid - found in most vegetables, fruits, and herbs; but most abundantly in the bark of willow trees, from where it was extracted for use in the early manufacture of aspirin.

Other nonflavonoid phenolics

- Curcumin - Curcumin has low bioavailability, because, much of it is excreted through glucuronidation. However, bioavailability is substantially enhanced by solubilization in a lipid (oil or lecithin), heat, addition of piperine, or through nano-particularization.
- Flavonolignans - e.g. silymarin - a mixture of flavonolignans extracted from milk thistle.
- Xanthones - mangosteen is purported to contain a large variety of xanthones, but some of the xanthones like mangostin might be present only in the inedible shell.
- Eugenol

Other potential organic antioxidants

- Capsaicin, the active component of chili peppers
- Bilirubin, a breakdown product of blood, has been identified as a possible antioxidant.
- Citric acid, oxalic acid, and phytic acid
- N-Acetylcysteine, water soluble
- R-α-Lipoic acid, fat and water soluble

Survey of antioxidant capacity of blueberry, blackberry, and strawberry (Huang et al, 2012)

Berries are a good source of natural antioxidants. In the present study, the total antioxidant capacity and phenolic composition of three berry fruits (blueberry, blackberry, and strawberry) cultivated in Nanjing were investigated.

Blueberry, with a Trolox equivalent antioxidant capacity (TEAC) value of 14.98 mmol Trolox/100 g dry weight (DW), **exhibited the strongest total antioxidant capacity using both the 2,2-azinobis(3-ethylbenzothiazoline-6-sulfonic acid) diammonium salt (ABTS) and the 2,2-diphenyl-1-picrylhydrazyl (DPPH) methods.**

Blueberry also had the highest total phenolic content (TPC, 9.44 mg gallic acid/g DW), total flavonoid content (TFC, 36.08 mg rutin/g DW), and total anthocyanidin content (TAC, 24.38 mg catechin/g DW).

A preliminary analysis using high performance liquid chromatography (HPLC) showed that the blueberry, blackberry, and strawberry samples tested contained a range of phenolic acids (including gallic acid, protocatechuic acid, p-hydroxybenzoic acid, vanillic acid, caffeic acid, p-coumaric acid, ferulic acid, ellagic acid, and cinnamic acid) and various types of flavonoids (flavone: luteolin; flavonols: rutin, myricetin, quercetrin, and quercetin; flavanols: gallocatechin, epigallocatechin, catechin, and catechin gallate; anthocyanidins: malvidin-3-galactoside, malvidin-3-glucoside, and cyanidin). In particular, **the blueberries had high levels of proanthocyanidins and anthocyanidins, which might be responsible for their strong antioxidant activities *in vitro*.**

These results indicate a potential market role for berries (especially blueberries) as a functional food ingredient or nutraceutical. (Huang et al, 2012)

Antioxidants were thought to be highly effective in the management of ROS-mediated tissue impairments (EMODs). Many antioxidant compounds possess anti-inflammatory, antiatherosclerotic, antiproliferative, antitumor, antimutagenic, anticarcinogenic, antibacterial, or antiviral activities to a greater or lesser extent. (Liu et al, 2002)

Berries (e.g., blueberry, blackberry, and strawberry) are well known as so-called "super fruits" for their potential in the nutraceutical and functional food markets. (Ding et al, 2006) (Tulipani et al, 2008)

RMH Note: There are no "super foods," none, zippo, nada!

Blueberries are flowering plants of the genus *Vaccinium* with dark-purple berries, **whose anthocyanins are considered to be nature's most potent antioxidants** and have demonstrated properties that extend well beyond suppressing free radicals. (Srivastava et al, 2007) (Srivastava A, Akoh CC, Fischer J, Krewer G. Effect of anthocyanin fractions from selected cultivars of Georgia-grown blueberries on apoptosis and phase II enzymes. J Agric Food Chem.2007;55(8):3180–3185)

Consumption of blueberries **may** alleviate the cognitive decline occurring in Alzheimer's disease and other conditions of aging. (Krikorian et al, 2010)

Allegedly, **blueberries also help maintain healthy blood flow via several mechanisms including healthy low-density lipoprotein (LDL) oxidation, normal platelet aggregation, and maintenance of endothelial function**. (Kalt et al, 2008) (Shaughnessy et al, 2009)

Blackberries are aggregate fruits produced by several species in the genus *Rubus* (e.g., *R. fruticosus*, *R. ursinus*, and *R. argutus*). **Blackberries are notable for their health benefits based on high nutritional contents of dietary fiber, vitamin C, vitamin K, folic acid, and the essential mineral, manganese.** (Sariburun et al, 2010)

Blackberries also rank highly among fruits for antioxidant strength, particularly due to their high contents of phenolic compounds, such as ellagic acid, tannins, ellagitannins, quercetin, gallic acid, anthocyanins, and cyanidins. (Hager et al, 2008)

Strawberries (*Fragaria x ananassa* Duch.) are widely appreciated for their excellent taste, characteristic aroma, and bright red color. Strawberries are an excellent source of vitamin C, and are also rich in bioactive phenolic compounds including flavonoids and phenolic acids, such as hydroxycinnamic acids, ellagic acids, ellagitannins, xavan-3-ols, xavonols, and anthocyanins.

Strawberries have been shown to have a remarkably high scavenging activity toward chemically generated radicals, thus making them effective in inhibiting oxidation of human LDLs. (Heinonen et al, 1998)

If the free radical theory had been proven true, the antioxidant activity of strawberries could contribute to the prevention of cancer, cardiovascular and other chronic diseases. (Hannum, 2004)

Because of their remarkable, *in vitro* antioxidant capacity, berries have received increasing attention in the past two decades, especially in North America and Europe.

A large number of studies on the physiological functions and chemical constituents of blueberry, blackberry, and strawberry have been reported. (Tulipani et al, 2008) (Krikorian et al, 2010)

Furthermore, no reports are available on the antioxidant capacity or detailed phenolic composition of blueberries, blackberries, or strawberries cultivated in Nanjing, China.

Reactive oxygen species (ROS), such as superoxide, hydrogen peroxide, and hydroxyl radicals, and free radical-meditated reactions, **may** cause oxidative damage to cellular structures and functional molecules (e.g., DNA, proteins, and lipids). (Finkel and Holbrook, 2000)

Older, discounted evidence suggested that oxidant stress is a major cause of many diseases, including aging, cancer, diabetes, cardiovascular disease, Alzheimer's disease, and other neurodegenerative disorders. (Halliwell, 1994)

CONCLUSIONS

Blueberries, blackberries, and strawberries cultivated in Nanjing exhibited potent antioxidant capacity and contained a variety of phenolic compounds. The results showed that the **blueberries had the strongest total antioxidant capacity, and also had the highest TPC, TFC, and TAC, when compared to blackberries and strawberries.**

The blueberries had particularly high levels of anthocyanidins and proanthocyanidins, which may be responsible for their very strong antioxidant activity. Therefore they may have potential for use in the development of nutraceuticals or as functional food ingredients of benefit to human health.

Human Effect Matrix For Blueberries

The following information was excerpted or modified from (Human Effect Matrix For Blueberries, 2013). This appears to be pro-blueberry article.

(Human Effect Matrix For Blueberries, 2013) (http://examine.com/supplements/Blueberry/)

Summary: My condensation for the educated consumer

- DNA damage appears to be acutely decreased following consumption of blueberries or its extracts (375mg anthocyanins or more) and tends to be in the range of a 20% reduction.

- Although the leaf extract has once been associated with a reduction in blood glucose, the fruits do not appear to inhibit carbohydrate absorption nor reduce fasting glucose.

- No known interactions with heart rate and blueberry supplementation.

- Blueberries do not appear to significantly influence nitric oxide metabolism.

- Supplementation of blueberry extract does appear effective in elderly persons with general cognitive decline, able to improve cognition and memory.

- Memory formation in elderly subjects can be improved with daily supplementation of blueberries or their extract.

- Insulin has once been noted to be decreased in elderly persons with blueberry ingestion.

- A slight improvement in subjective well being and happiness has been noted in elderly persons given blueberries over a few weeks as a daily supplement.

- Oral ingestion of berries or their extracts tends to reduce oxidative biomarkers and improve antioxidant status either acutely or with daily supplementation.

- There appears to be a reduction in LDL oxidation, with the one chronic study suggesting a 27% reduction (the acute study noting less of a protective effect).

- No significant influence on appetite or satiety.

- A decrease in blood pressure has been noted in persons at risk for cardiovascular disease (6% systolic and 4% diastolic), but this may be limited to high risk individuals only.

- No known interactions with serum triglycerides following supplementation of blueberries.

- C-reactive protein does not appear to be influenced with blueberry supplementation.

- No significant changes in TNF-alpha concentrations.

- No significant influence on total cholesterol concentrations in the blood.

- No significant changes in LDL-C concentrations in serum with blueberries.

- No significant influence on HDL-C.

- An improvement of insulin sensitivity has been noted in persons with insulin resistance, but this may only affect high risk individuals.

- Despite the reduction in muscle damage and increased rate of recovery, there are no significant changes in subjective muscle soreness.

- Appears to reduce biomarkers of muscle damage such as creatine kinase.

- No significant influence on IL-6 concentrations in serum.

- Exercise-induced changes in cortisol are not influence by blueberry supplementation.

- The study to measure nF-kB binding activity in muscle tissue after exercise failed to find an influence of blueberry supplementation.

- The lone study using a 2.5 hour running protocol at 72% VO2 max failed to find any significant differences between groups in oxidative status after exercise.

- An increase in IL-10 following exercise has been noted.

- An increase in natural killer cells has been noted in the range of 76-122% following physical exercise.

- The alterations in most immune cells seen during exercise are wholly unaffected by blueberry supplementation.

- Chronic loading of blueberries with an acute dose prior to prolonged exercise (2.5 hours) in trained men does not improve physical performance.

- Currently no studies noting changes in HbA1c, as it appears to be unaffected by supplementation.

- No significant influence on weight when taken as a daily supplement in obese individuals.

- Alongside the reduction in serum oxidation comes a reduction in lipid peroxidation biomarkers such as MDA.

- No significant alterations in cell adhesion factors (sCAM-1 and vCAM-1).

- No significant influence on adiponectin concentrations in obese individuals.

(Human Effect Matrix For Blueberries, 2013) (http://examine.com/supplements/Blueberry/)

Blueberries contain a lot of molecules called anthocyanins, which are claimed to improve cognition.

Blueberries are a small, blue-purple fruit that belong to the genus vaccinium, which also includes cranberries and bilberries.

Blueberries are a popular food and frequently supplemented. The antioxidant and anthocyanin content of blueberries makes them particularly exploitable in false claims for reducing cognitive decline, supporting cardiovascular health, protecting the liver, and reducing liver fat buildup.

Blueberries may also have a potential Nootropic effect. They have been found to improve cognition in people undergoing cognitive decline, but there is also some rodent evidence that suggests blueberries can improve cognition in healthy young people as well. They may also have a role to play in promoting the growth of nervous tissue and reducing neurological inflammation.

Blueberries can be supplemented through a blueberry extract, isolated anthocyanins, or frozen or fresh blueberries.

The optimal dose for blueberry extract is 5.5 – 11g, with the higher end of the dose being more effective. The optimal range for isolated anthocyanin supplementation is 500-1,000mg. The optimal dose for blueberry extract translates to approximately 60-120g of fresh berries.

Blueberries should be eaten or supplemented daily. They are best stored in cold environments, like a refrigerator. Blanching blueberries is known to increase anthocyanin bioavailability, but excessive heat treatment or exposure will degrade the anthocyanin content.

Studies that measure blueberry intake in rats tend to use dehydrated powders rather than blueberry fruits, and thus the weight is in reference to dry weight rather than wet weight

Blueberries can be eaten or supplemented through blueberry powder. Isolated anthocyanins are also an effective supplement. Blueberries are both a food product and dietary supplement.

The Human Matrix attempts to show the effects of blueberries in humans, but many rodent studies are included.

Sources and Composition

Vaccinium (of the family *Ericaceae*) is a genus of berry making plants which contain a few common classes of berries, with the particular section of this genus (*Vaccinium cyanococcus*) being those plants which bear blueberries. There are several species of plants which bear blueberries, including:

- Rabbiteye blueberry (*Vaccinium ashei* and *Vaccinium virgatum* are both called this)
- Lowbush blueberry (*Vaccinium angustifolium*)
- Northern highbush blueberry (*Vaccinium corymbosum*)
- Wild Bog blueberry (*Vaccinium uliginosum*)
- Andean blueberry (*Vaccinium floribundu*)
- Colombian blueberry (*Vaccinium meridionale*)

Other sections include the European blueberry or 'Bilberry' (*Vaccinium myrtillus*]), Natsuhaze (*Vaccinium oldhamii*), Shashanbo (*Vaccinium bracteatum*), and cranberries (*Vaccinium oxycoccus*, of which oxycoccus refers to a subgenus), while some other berries that just happen to be blue-ish in color sometimes falsely carry the blueberry name such as neotropical blueberry (*Anthopterus wardii*).

Blueberries are known to have a high anthocyanin content which confers relatively potent antioxidant potential which has been noted to collectively confer about 85% of total antioxidant capacities of blueberries (the rest coming from other flavonoids). (Borges et al, 2010) (Borges G, *et al*. Identification of flavonoid and phenolic antioxidants in black currants, blueberries, raspberries, red currants, and cranberries. *J Agric Food Chem*. (2010)

The fruits themselves (not dehydrated powder) tend to have a 201.4-402.8mg/100g range (0.2-0.4%) of anthocyanins, **they are mostly rich in the two anthocyanins: malvidin and delphinidin.**

The anthocyanins seem to be stored in the peels (693-8814.9mg/100g dry weight) to a larger degree than the fruit (93.8-528.6mg/100g), and correlate with color of the berries (**the darker blue-purple being associated with more anthocyanins**).

Structure

Anthocyanins are a class of bioflavonoid which are characterized by having a 2-phenylbenzopyrylium (flavylium cation) skeleton with added hydroxyl or methoxy groups. Relative to other flavonoids, they are different as the oxygen in their backbone is highly polar.

The term procyanidin (interchangeable with 'proanthocyanidin') is used to refer to dimers or larger compounds composed of catechin molecules; commonly seen in food products or supplements that also have a catechin content such as Cocoa Extract, Grape Seed Extract, or Pycnogenol.

Despite being named proanthocyanidins, they have no relation to the anthocyanins.

Properties

Freeze drying has been found to reduce total anthocyanin content by 3.9%, which is not an overly large amount as anthocyanins can inherently vary two-fold in blueberries. Various phenolics acids (ferulic, vanillic, etc.) experience a 1.9-fold increase upon freezing.

Blanching berries (usually prior to processing) does not appear to inherently alter anthocyanin content (increase in the content of chlorogenic acid and other phenolic acids)[39] and may reduce the losses in other forms of treatment. Furthermore, blanched berry products appear to have a 25% increased bioavailability of anthocyanins when compared to control berries.

Heat treatment of anthocyanin containing berries (as puree) for 20 minutes as increasing temperatures (20-70°C range) is able to reduce anthocyanin count by 21%.

Refrigeration of heat-treated anthocyanins results in degradation, with 60 days of storage at 31°C causing complete elimination of anthocyanins (despite other polyphenolics being preserved).

In cold storage, blueberries are either stable or experience small increases in anthocyanin content and total antioxidant capacity.

Exposure to high oxygen environments does not appear to negatively affect the anthocyanin content of blueberries, instead, they curiously caused a slight increase. (Zheng et al, 2003)

Fruits versus Supplementation

It has been noted that an oral intake of approximately 2% blueberry lyophilized powder in the diet of rats (which is about 400mg per rat or 1g/kg) is equivalent to oral intake of 0.16g/kg in humans or, for a 150lb human, 10.9g. As 400mg blueberry powder is equivalent to 4,400mg fresh blueberries (water weight inclusive), then 10.9g of the powder is approximately 120g of blueberries.

Longevity

Caloric Restriction

Dietary supplementation of polyphenolics (a mixture of blueberry at 2%, pomegranate at 0.3%, and the Green Tea Catechins EGCG at 155mcg/kg) alongside caloric restriction **appears to augment the pro-longevity effects of said caloric restriction** (enhancing the median lifespan from a 37% increase to a 46%) which was hypothesized to be due to the polyphenolics suppressing neuronal inflammation which was unregulated in caloric restriction control. (Aires et al, 2012)

Pharmacology

Digestion and Absorption

Anthocyanins appear to undergo slightly degradation in saliva (with aglycones being more susceptible than glycosides), which appears to be mediated by salivary bacteria.

The bioavailability of anthocyanins (regardless of source) tends to be in the range of 1.7-3.3%.

Serum

Anthocyanins have been confirmed to be absorbed from the intestines and oral ingestion of 720mg anthocyanins (as glycosides) in older women has been noted to increase serum anthocyanins to 97.4nM. **RMH Note: These nanomolar levels are still extremely low**.

In otherwise healthy men consuming 300mg fresh berries (348mg anthocyanins), plasma anthocyanins have been noted to reach 13.7+/-10.7nM after one hour and 18.7+/-6.4nM after two hours.

Blueberry juice consumption (1,000mL) has also been confirmed to be a bioavailable source of Quercetin.

Metabolism

Blueberry tannin structures have been noted to be metabolized into smaller phenolic acids via the bacteria *Lactobacillus plantarum* (expresses tannase) such as phenyllactic acid, hydroxylactic acid, and 3,4-dihydroxyphenylpropionic acid. This bacteria is found in a variety of fermented food products, and can survive in the human intestinal tract and thus these metabolites may be biologically relevant.

Neurology

Glutaminergic Neurotransmission

NDMA receptor dependent long term potentiation (LTP) is a process that is known to be involved in memory formation and its decline with aging known to (in part) underlie memory loss, particularly spatial memory formation. This hypoactivity is thought to be due to both less receptor expression and less stimuli to activate signaling.

Supplementation of 1.8% blueberry water extract in the diet of aged **rats** over eight weeks is able to restore LTP in the hippocampus back to the level of young control rats although **it did not appear to restore levels of the** NMDA receptor subunits that were impaired in aged rats, although it could increase NR2B phosphorylation. (Coultrap et al, 2008)

Appetite

In diabetic rats, supplementation of blueberry juice appears to attenuate the diabetes-induced hyperphagia (which resulted in less weight gained). **Other studies using rats and blueberries in the dosage range of 1-3% do not find significant alterations in food intake.** (Yuji et al, 2013)

The addition of 50g fresh blueberries to a test meal has failed to significantly alter the satiety rating of the meal in humans. (Clegg et al, 2011)

The lone human study using 50g of blueberries alongside a meal failed to find an effect.

Neuroinflammation

In vitro, blueberries have shown anti-inflammatory effects via reducing the release of inflammatory biomarkers (TNF-α and COX2) from activated microglia, which respond to inflammatory signals and contribute to some pathological conditions of cognitive decline.

In cells exposed to TNF-α (proinflammatory molecule that can cause oxidation via NADPH oxidase activation from sphingolipids), **5µg/mL of blueberry extract can reduce oxidation to near control levels without affecting basal oxidation *in vitro*;** this is thought to be due to inhibiting the NADPH oxidase enzyme from assembling in the plasma membranes which is required for NADPH oxidase functioning.

Neurogenesis

Blueberry ingestion has been noted to augment a kainic acid induced increase in IGF-1 at 2% of the diet over 8 weeks, without inherent effect on **rats** not administrated kainic acid. (Shukitt-Hale et al, 2008)
Dietary supplementation of 2% blueberry (179.0mcg/g anthocyanins and 74.1mcg/g flavanols) as well as either the anthocyanins or flavanols in isolation at the same dose was able to increase brain BDNF levels with no influence on pro-BDNF, and the anthocyanin group increased BDNF mRNA levels (81% in the hippocampus). This has been confirmed to occur in otherwise healthy young rats as well at 2% of the diet as blueberries.

Memory and Learning

Isolated Pterostilbene has been noted to improve cognition in **aged rats** when fed in the diet at 0.004-0.016% over 12-13 weeks, with the improvements correlating with hippocampal concentrations of pterostilbene. **Similar benefits have been found with 2% blueberries in the diet, although this study attributed the observed benefit to anthocyanins.** (Andres-Lacueva et al, 2005)

Cognitive impairments by kainic acid as assessed by water maze have been noted to be attenuated with 2% blueberry in the diet over 8 weeks in rats and the cognitive decline (object recognition task) in aged rats appears to be normalized to young control at the same dose.

In aged rats given 2% blueberries or the anthocyanin equivalent (179mcg/g), the improvements in spatial memory and attention performance were increased to an equal degree.

In studies on cognitive decline in rats, the addition of either blueberries to the diet or isolated blueberry components is able to reverse or at least attenuate the changes seen in cognition.

An improvement in spatial memory formation has been confirmed in otherwise healthy young rats given blueberry daily.

In twelve elderly humans (an extremely small study group) with age-related memory decline, concord grape juice (6-9mL/kg, anthocyanin content not disclosed) daily for 12 weeks was **associated with an improvement of verbal learning with nonsignificant benefits in spatial and verbal recall** and a later study using similar dosing in a similar population found cognitive benefit with wild blueberry juice (428-598mg anthocyanins daily) as assessed by verbal memory tests. (Krikorian et al, 2010, BJNutr)

Anthocyanins as well as blueberry juice itself have been demonstrated to improve cognition in elderly humans.

Cardiovascular Health

Cardiac Tissue

A higher dietary intake of anthocyanins is associated with less risk for myocardial infarction in young and middle-aged women. (Cassidy et al, 2013)

There appears to be a protective effect on cardiac lesions induced by myocardial infarction when blueberry is supplemented at 2% of the **rat** diet for three months preceding experimental infarction. (Ahmet et al, 2009)

One year of daily blueberry supplementation at 2% of the **rat** diet *following* an experimental myocardial infarction showed protective effects as mortality was reduced by 22% in the blueberry group relative to placebo without influencing blood pressure nor heart rate.

It appears that blueberry supplementation causes an increase in the threshold required for mitochondrial permeability transition (MTPt) to around 24% at 2% of the diet. MTP is increased by reactive oxygen species and involved in increasing mitochondrial permeability and cell death by causing an influx of molecules into the mitochondria, and the increased threshold seen with blueberry ingestion makes it more difficult for a stressor to cause cell death via MTP.

Blood Flow and Pressure

In **rats** fed blueberries (fermented with *Lactobacillus plantarum* to break down tannins into smaller compounds) or the isolated molecules that were produced after fermentation (phenylactic acid, hydroxylactic acid, and 3,4-dihydroxyphenylpropionic acid) **failed to reduce the hypertension caused by L-NAME**. (Xu et al, 2013)

Elsewhere, **blueberries have been found to reduce blood pressure in hypertensive rats (spontaneously hypertensive rats) at 2-3% of the diet** which has been replicated elsewhere. (Elks et al, 2011) (Shaughnessy et al, 2009)

300g fresh berries (348mg anthocyanins) has failed to influence blood flow, heart rate, or nitric oxide concentrations following acute administration. (Del Bo et al, 2013)
In persons at risk for cardiovascular disease, 50g of freeze dried blueberries (350g berry equivalent; 1624mg phenolics and 742mg anthocyanins) daily for eight weeks **is able to reduce both systolic (6%) and diastolic (4%) blood pressure.** (Basu et al, 2010)

Lipoproteins

Anthocyanins appear to be able to prevent the oxidation of LDL cholesterol *in vitro* with malvidin being the most potent anthocyanin yet blackberries being more potent than blueberries (despite the high malvidin percentage of the latter) due to more overall anthocyanins.

Oral ingestion of 75g of fresh berries (1.3% anthocyanins) alongside a standardized meal has been noted to delay lipoprotein oxidation *in vivo* when measured at three hours after the meal and in persons at risk for cardiovascular disease daily intake of 742mg anthocyanins over eight weeks is associated with a 27% reduction in LDL oxidation.

Oral consumption of 22.5g blueberry extract (1462mg phenolics and 668mg anthocyanins) daily for six weeks in obese and insulin resistant persons **failed to significantly alter HDL-C, LDL-C, or total cholesterol and these lipid biomarkers are unaffected with 724mg of anthocyanins daily for eight weeks in persons at risk for cardiovascular disease.** (Basu et al, 2010)

Triglycerides

In guinea pigs fed a high cholesterol diet and 8% blueberries by weight, blueberry ingestion failed to influence serum triglycerides despite reducing hepatic triglycerides (50% attenuation). (Coban et al, 2013)

This inefficacy of blueberries on serum triglycerides extends to other animals such as rats.

Oral consumption of blueberry (1462mg phenolics and 668mg anthocyanins) over six weeks in obese and insulin resistant persons has failed to reduce triglycerides and in persons at risk for cardiovascular disease there is still no change in triglycerides. (Stull et al, 2010) (Basu et al, 2010)

Artherosclerosis

Ingestion of 1% of the mouse diet as blueberries appears to be able to delay progression of artherosclerotic lesions in ApoE$^{-/-}$ mice without apparent changes in lipoprotein and triglyceride levels. (Wu et al, 2010)

Interactions with Glucose Metabolism

Carbohydrate Absorption

Isolated components of blueberries have previously been linked to inhibiting enzymes of carbohydrate absorption.

The potency of blueberries seem less than that of red berries, apparently due to the soluble tannin component.

Oral ingestion of 50g fresh blueberries mixed into pancakes (compared to control pancakes) failed to significantly affect postprandial glucose absorption (both max value and AUC were unaltered). (Clegg et al, 2011)

High dose anthocyanin supplementation (100g berries conferring 1,200mg anthocyanins) has failed to reduce the postprandial spike in blood glucose, instead being associated with a slight increase 3-4 hours after ingestion. (Kay, Holub, 2002)

Blood glucose

While one study using blueberry leaves (50mg Myricetin and 50mg Chlorogenic Acid per 300mg supplemental leaf extract) in type II diabetics has reported a reduction in blood glucose from 143+/-5.2mg/L to 104+/-5.7mg/L (28%), **other studies using blueberry fruits have failed to note reductions in blood glucose in persons with insulin resistance or persons at risk for cardiovascular disease.** (Basu et al, 2010)

Insulin Sensitivity

Consumption of 22.5g blueberry extract (1462mg phenolics and 668mg anthocyanins) daily for six weeks in obese but non-diabetic adults with insulin resistance was able to improve insulin sensitivity by more than 10% in two-thirds of participants, with an average group mean improvement of 22.2+/-5.8% (placebo 4.9+/-4.5%).

A failure to benefit insulin sensitivity has been noted elsewhere in persons who were not insulin resistant. (Basu et al, 2010)

Fat Mass and Obesity

Mechanisms

In rat adipocytes (3T3-F442A), 150-250mg/mL of blueberry polyphenols is able to suppress the differentiation of fat cells and dose-dependently reduce lipid accumulation (27-74%).

Blueberry polyphenols at doses of up to 250mg/mL have failed to significantly increase lipolysis. (Moghe et al, 2012)

Interventions

Blueberry appears to be able to improve glucose tolerance and handling in the body, and even in interventions where weight is loss (naturally aids in glucose tolerance) it cannot fully explain the actions of blueberries.

Despite apparent improvements in insulin sensitivity, weight gain and fat cell size as well as adipokines (leptin and adiponectin) are not affected by blueberry supplementation. (DeFuria et al, 2009)

Although there have been failures for the fruit extracts themselves to reduce fat mass there are some studies noting efficacy; it is unsure what underlies the differences in the observed results.

When looking at interventions measuring fat gain over time, blueberry juice and purified anthocyanins appear to exert a minor anti-obese effect, which is less reliably seen with the whole fruits.

Exercise and Skeletal Muscle

Interventions

Consumption of blueberries in a smoothie 10 and 5 hours before exercise (as well as immediately after and 12 and 36 hours afterwards; five drinks in total with each consisting of 200g berries and 96.6mg anthocyanins) **is able to speed up the recovery of power following eccentric leg extensions, but does not appear to influence muscle soreness nor fatigue during the workout.** (McLeay et al, 2012)

Skeleton and Bone Mass

Consumption of blueberries in the diet of pre-pubertal female rats was effective in preventing menopausal bone loss later in life, despite supplementation not continuing for that time.[121]

Interactions with Oxidation

Mechanisms

Anthocyanins have been noted to directly sequester superoxide radicals, hydroxyl radicals, lipid peroxides and lipid peroxidation induced by copper, and the nitric oxide free radical.

This antioxidant capacity of blueberries appears to occur intracellularly at very low concentrations (less than 1µg/mL anthocyanin concentration) which suggests that they are active despite the poor oral absorption. **RMH Note: remember that anthocyanins only reach nano-molar levels.**

Ingestion of blueberries (35g or 75g fresh berries) alongside breakfast noted that the higher dose was associated with a higher plasma antioxidant capacity as well as increased urate and Vitamin C concentrations.

The actions of the enzyme NADPH oxidase require it to gather in the membrane of a cell where it localizes with its subunits, and then it can produce superoxide radicals and contribute to oxidation.

Blueberries have been noted to inhibit the NADPH oxidase enzyme, and a fraction of the berry that is nonpolar (not anthocyanins) appears to be able to do this despite having a poor direct antioxidative effect.

Some believe that blueberries may inhibit NADPH oxidase, which would reduce the oxidation produced from an overactive immune system.

Antioxidant Enzymes

Antioxidant enzymes including SOD, Glutathione peroxidase, and catalase (reduced by DMBA toxin) **have been noted to be preserved with blueberry** (200mg/kg) and the reduction seen in hepatic fibrosis also abrogated. (Kavitha et al, 2013)

This may be another way to produce antioxidant capacity.

Irradiation

75µg/mL of blueberry anthocyanins or procyanidins have both been shown to reduce UV-induced DNA damage in cellular cultures. (Liu et al, 2013)

DNA Repair

DNA repair enzymes have been noted to be upregulated with blueberry extract (200mg/kg), with a potency greater than Astaxanthin (15mg/kg) and ellagic acid (0.4mg/kg) but lesser than chlorophyllin (4mg/kg).

DNA damage has been noted to be reduced in humans following consumption of blueberry extract (15g powder conferring 375mg anthocyanins) for six weeks as assessed by less formamidopyrimidine DNA glycosylase (FPG)–sensitive sites (24.2%) and **H_2O_2 induced damage (19.8%) and over four weeks of 1,000mL of a blueberry drink DNA damage has been noted to be reduced in healthy controls** (20% less oxidative damage).

Following **acute oral ingestion of 300g fresh blueberries** (348mg anthocyanins and 727mg phenolic acids) **to otherwise healthy male subjects in the form of a gel (in order to mask placebo) noted that a single oral dose of blueberries was able to reduce H_2O_2 induced DNA damage from 51.7% to 42.7%.** (Del Bo et al, 2013)

However, the reduced DNA damage was very transient and disappeared after two hours and other studies using 200g of a mixed berry desert daily for two weeks have failed to find a significant change in basal DNA damage. (Carmen-Ramirez-Tortosa et al, 2004)

This may not be of advantage since it is so short lived.

Inflammation and Immunology

Virology

The phenolics of blueberries may possess anti-influenza properties *in vitro*. (Sekizawa et al, 2013)

Exercise Immunology

Oral ingestion of 250g fresh berries daily for six weeks (and a single dose of 375g taken one hour before exercise) in well trained runners subject to 2.5 hours of moderate intensity exercise (72% VO_2 max) is able to **increase serum IL-10** relative to control and increase natural killer cell count by 76-122%, although **other immune cells (leukocytes, neutrophils, monocytes, and both T and B lymphocytes) and cytokines (IL-1ra, IL-6, IL-8) were unaffected.** (McAnulty et al, 2011)

Interactions with Organ Systems

Liver

In studies assessing liver fat, oral supplementation of blueberries to the diets of rats appears to cause a dose-dependent reduction in hepatic fat accumulation.

Reductions in liver fat can occur independently of any changes in serum triglyceride, which blueberry supplementation does not appear to significantly influence.

The oxidative stress induced by diethylnitrosamine is able to be attenuated with high dose blueberry supplementation in rats (5-10% of the diet) and **blueberry juice has been noted to reduce fibrosis induced by CCL$_4$** over 8 weeks when consumed at 15g/kg daily. (Bingul et al, 2013) (Wang et al, 2013)

Kidneys

Supplementation of 2% blueberries in the diets of hypertensive rats is able to improve glomerular filtration rate and reduce renovascular resistance secondary to improving blood pressure; these changes are thought to be due to antioxidant properties of the blueberries as improvements in oxidative biomarkers in the kidneys were noted.

Nutrient-Nutrient Interactions

Spirulina

Spirulina is a highly efficacious antioxidant compound due to the C-phycocyanin component, with 0.1-0.33% of the diet as spirulina being more neuroprotective than a diet of 2% blueberries acutely albeit the opposite trend at 4 weeks afterwards.

NT-020 is a combination of polyphenols from blueberry, Green Tea Catechins, carnosine (from Beta-Alanine) and Vitamin D and **this combination supplement appears to be synergistic with Spirulina in enhancing stem cell proliferation** (CD34+ derived bone marrow cells). NT-020 overall is known to do this in a synergistic manner itself with all bioactives being somewhat active (hypothesized to be secondary to reducing oxidative stress).

Vinegar

Blueberries fermented in Alcohol followed shortly by acetic acid fermentation (**vinegar, which is also inherently bioactive**) resulting **in a fruit vinegar of 5.6% blueberry and 59.14% acetic acid failed to activate hepatic genes involved in fat metabolism** (PPARα, CPT-1 and ACO) despite pomegranate vinegar doing so. This synergism was thought to be due to the ellagic acid and Punicalagins content, both of which are not present in blueberries. (Kim et al, 2013)

Berries: emerging impact on cardiovascular health

The following information was excerpted or modified from (Basu et al, 2010).

Berries are a good source of polyphenols, especially anthocyanins, micronutrients, and fiber. In epidemiological and clinical studies, these constituents have been associated with improved cardiovascular risk profiles.

Human intervention studies using chokeberries, cranberries, blueberries, and strawberries (either fresh, or as juice, or freeze-dried), or purified anthocyanin extracts have demonstrated significant improvements in LDL oxidation, lipid peroxidation, total plasma antioxidant capacity, dyslipidemia, and glucose metabolism. Benefits were seen in healthy subjects and in those with existing metabolic risk factors. (Basu et al, 2010)

Consumption of fruits and vegetables has been correlated with decreased risks of cardiovascular disease (CVD). National health objectives reflected in *Healthy People 2010* advocate increasing fruit consumption by more than 75% or to at least two servings per day in persons 2 years of age and older. Currently, only 32% of adults and 13% of adolescents meet this goal of fruit intake.

The commonly consumed berries in the United States include blackberry, black raspberry, blueberry, cranberry, red raspberry, and strawberries. Less commonly consumed berries include acai, black currant, chokeberry, and mulberries.

Berries are low in calories and are high in moisture and fiber.

They contain natural antioxidants such as vitamins C and E, and micronutrients such as folic acid, calcium, selenium, alpha and beta carotene, and lutein.

Phytochemicals found in berries include polyphenols along with high proportions of flavonoids including anthocyanins and ellagitannins.

Anthocyanins comprise the largest group of natural, water-soluble, plant pigments and impart the bright colors to berry fruits and to flowers.

Approximately 400 individual anthocyanins have been determined.

They are generally more concentrated in the skins of fruits, especially berry fruits. However, red berry fruits, such as strawberries and cherries, also have anthocyanins in their flesh. Anthocyanin content is usually proportional to the color intensity and can range from 2 to 4 g/kg, increasing as the fruit ripens.

Evidence suggests that Americans consume an average of 12.5–215 mg of anthocyanins per day.

Studies have shown that berry anthocyanins are poorly bioavailable, are extensively conjugated in the intestines and liver, and are excreted in urine within 2–8 hours post consumption. (Kroon et al, 2004) (Netzel et al, 2002) **RMH Note: Lack of bioavailability is very important to keep in mind when evaluating clinical human studies.**

Post-harvest processing, such as pressing, pasteurization, and conventional and vacuum drying, can significantly affect the polyphenol (including anthocyanin) and vitamin content of berries, and therefore their bioactivities. (Srivastava et al, 2007) (Hartmann et al, 2008) (Wojdylo et al, 2009)

Nutritional epidemiology provides convincing evidence of the cardioprotective effects of frequent consumption of fruits and vegetables high in fiber, micronutrients, and several phytochemicals. Data reported from the INTERHEART study, comprising dietary patterns from 52 countries, revealed a significant inverse association between the prudent dietary pattern high in fruits and vegetables, and risk of acute myocardial infarction. (Iqbal et al, 2008)

A comparative study between the US and French populations revealed significantly lower fruit and vegetable consumption among American men and women versus French adults. Analyses of 24-h recall data from the National Health and Nutrition Examination Survey (NHANES), 1999–2000, revealed that **only 40% of Americans consumed five or more servings of fruits and vegetables per day.** (Guenther et al, 2006)

NHANES (2001–2002) data reported the pattern of fruit intake among US adults, who mainly consumed apples, pears, and bananas, followed by melons, citrus fruits, and grapes. Thus, **berries do not seem to be commonly consumed fruits by the US population in spite of**

their benefits, as documented in emerging nutrition and health research. (Bachman et al, 2008)

Studies have also reported specific associations between berries or berry flavonoids (anthocyanins) and cardiovascular health. Data reported from **the Kuopio Ischemic Heart Disease Risk Factor Study (KIHD) showed a significantly lower risk of CVD-related deaths among 1,950 men in the highest quartile of berry intake** (>408 g/day) versus men with the lowest intake (<133 g/day) during a mean follow-up of 12.8 years.

Post-menopausal women (*n* = 34,489) participating in **the Iowa Women's Health Study, showed a significant reduction in CVD mortality associated with strawberry intake during a 16-year follow-up period.**

In the case of blueberries, an age- and energy-adjusted model showed a significant decrease in coronary heart disease mortality, though the significance did not persist following adjustment for other confounding variables. For both strawberries and blueberries, the significant reduction in relative risk was associated with at least once per week consumption. The data also reported that **a mean anthocyanin intake of 0.2 mg/day was associated with a significantly reduced risk of CVD mortality in these post-menopausal women.** (Mink et al, 2007)

Female US health professionals enrolled in **the Women's Health Study** (*n* = 38,176), a randomized controlled trial of low-dose aspirin and vitamin E, provided dietary information using a 131-item validated semi-quantitative food frequency questionnaire. Strawberry intake was described as "never" or "less than one serving per month" up to "6+ servings per day" of fresh, frozen, or canned strawberries. Analyses of baseline strawberry intake revealed that only 7.7% of subjects consumed greater than two servings of strawberries per week, whereas 42% of subjects reported an intake of 1–3 servings per month. During a follow-up period of approximately 11 years, a decreasing trend for CVD was observed for subjects consuming higher amounts of strawberries. The study also showed a borderline significant risk reduction of elevated C-reactive protein (CRP) levels (≥3 mg/L) among women consuming higher amounts of strawberries (≥2 servings/week).

Blueberry intake was also examined in the study and no significant association was reported with risks of CVD or CRP. (Sesso et al, 2007)

Elevated CRP has been significantly associated with inflammation and is a high risk factor of CVD. Analyses of NHANES data (1999–2002) revealed **a significant inverse association between serum CRP and anthocyanin intakes among US adults**. (Chun et al, 2008)

These observational data suggest a potential anti-inflammatory role of berry flavonoids, which may contribute to overall reduction of CVD risk.

Berries were also shown to increase plasma antioxidant capacity and to decrease lipid peroxidation in smokers who are at high risk of developing CVD.

Of 20 trials conducted using different varieties of fresh and processed berry products, **only two showed a significant decrease in systolic blood pressure: one was conducted in healthy men following cranberry juice supplementation and the other was in subjects with CVD risk factors following mixed berry supplementation.** (Ruel et al, 2008) (Erlund et al, 2008) (Erlund I, Koli R, Alfthan G, et al. Favorable effects of berry consumption on platelet function, blood pressure, and HDL cholesterol. Am J Clin Nutr. 2008;87:323–331)

Interestingly, **none of these clinical studies showed any significant effect of berry intervention on biomarkers of inflammation**, with the exception of a significant decrease in adhesion molecules following cranberry juice supplementation in healthy volunteers. (Ruel et al, 2008)

Anthocyanins from berries commonly consumed in the United States, such as blueberries and cranberries, have been reported to reduce TNF-α induced upregulation of inflammatory mediators in human microvascular endothelial cells. In an 8-week study, DeFuria et al. have shown **the attenuation of inflammatory gene expressions** in male C57Bl/6j mice fed a high-fat diet supplemented with blueberry powder versus the unsupplemented group. This study also showed **the protective effects of blueberries against insulin resistance and hyperglycemia, thus reducing the risk factors for CVD**. (DeFuria et al, 2009)

Purified anthocyanins from blueberries and strawberries added to drinking water were shown to prevent the development of dyslipidemia and obesity in mice fed a high-fat diet for a period of 90 days. (Prior et al, 2009)

Conclusion

While limited epidemiological data inversely associate consumption of berries with inflammation and CVD, these conclusions need to be strengthened in future case-control or cohort studies investigating the long-term health benefits of berries in specific populations.

Clinical studies in healthy humans, subjects with diabetes mellitus, dyslipidemia, metabolic syndrome, hypertension, or in smokers, show a significant decrease in CVD risk factors, especially glucose, lipids and lipid peroxidation, and systolic blood pressure, following berry intervention. (Basu et al, 2010)

In light of the decrease in nutritional value that occurs during processing methods, including drying and pasteurization, consumption of fresh or frozen whole berries as part of a regular diet may be better than intake of juices or extracts, which do not have the same nutritional profiles as whole berries. (Basu et al, 2010)

Blueberry effect on eccentric exercise-induced muscle damage

Exercise-induced muscle damage (EIMD) is accompanied by localized oxidative stress / inflammation which, in the short-term at least, is associated with impaired muscular performance. Dietary antioxidants have been shown to reduce excessive oxidative stress; however, **their effectiveness in facilitating recovery following EIMD is not clear**.

Blueberries demonstrate antioxidant and anti-inflammatory properties.

In a randomized cross-over design, 10 females consumed a blueberry smoothie or placebo of a similar antioxidant capacity 5 and 10 hours prior to and then immediately, 12 and 36 hours after EIMD induced by 300 strenuous eccentric contractions of the quadriceps. Blood biomarkers of oxidative stress, antioxidant capacity, and inflammation were assessed at 12, 36 and 60 hours post exercise. Data were analyzed using a two-way ANOVA. (McLeay et al, 2012)

Although a faster rate of decrease in oxidative stress was observed in the blueberry group, it was not significant ($p < 0.05$)

until 36 hours post-exercise and interestingly coincided with a gradual increase in plasma antioxidant capacity, whereas biomarkers for inflammation were still elevated after 60 hours recovery. This study demonstrates that the ingestion of a blueberry smoothie prior to and after EIMD accelerates recovery of muscle peak isometric strength. (McLeay et al, 2012)

Although **the mechanisms behind exercise-induced muscle damage (EIMD) are not precisely known** it is believed that along with initial mechanically-induced disruption of the extracellular matrix, sarcolemma, sarcoplasmic reticulum, t-tubules and contractile proteins, secondary damage is caused by the production of reactive oxygen species (ROS) at the site of injury by phagocytic cells. (Charge, Rudnicki, 2004)

While it is well understood that antioxidants play a pivotal role in countering free radical activity within the body, **research investigating classical antioxidant supplementation (such as vitamin C and E) on the rate of recovery from EIMD, particularly functional recovery, has consistently shown little or no benefit from supplementation**. (Goldfarb et al, 2011) (McGinley, Shafat, 2009) (Nieman, Stear, 2010)

Blueberry fruit are normally consumed as a whole fruit (fresh or frozen) and although they are low in vitamin C and E, **they contain the broadest range of anthocyanin and polyphenolic antioxidant compounds among common berry fruits**. (Wu et al, 2004)

Blueberry fruit exhibit a high antioxidant capacity (oxygen radical absorption capacity - ORAC) and have been shown to reduce oxidative stress and inflammation, indicating that blueberry-derived anthocyanins may modulate cellular events independent of the fruit's inherent antioxidant capacity. (McAnulty et al, 2004) (Hurst et al, 2010)

In this study we observed a rapid decline in oxidative stress blood indices that coincided with the increase in plasma antioxidant capacity in the blueberry condition supporting the notion that an increase in plasma antioxidant capacity may be involved in the reduced exercise-induced oxidative stress observed. However, **it is currently unclear whether an increase in plasma antioxidant capacity facilitates or hinders the activation of muscle adaptive events aiding muscle recovery**. (Theodorou et al, 2011)

Prof Randolph M Howes MD,PhD

The efficacy of dietary antioxidant supplementation in facilitating recovery following strenuous muscle damaging exercise is under debate. Recent reports indicate that dietary supplements rich in antioxidants, attenuate oxidative stress, whilst **other reports either show that antioxidants have no action or have the ability to induce pro-oxidant effects**. (Yfanti et al, 2010) (McAnulty et la, 2005) (Nieman et al, 2004)

Moreover, although elevated plasma antioxidant capacity post antioxidant supplementation consumption has been found in many studies **they have failed to demonstrate an effect or relationship to muscle function recovery following an eccentric exercise-induced damage.**
(Warren et al, 1992

Goldfarb *et al.* recently showed **that ingestion of whole fruit and/ or vegetable extracts may attenuate blood oxidative stress induced by eccentric exercise but no significant effect on functional changes relating to pain and muscle damage were observed.**
(Goldfarb et al, 2011)

Our findings here concur as **all correlations of indices of muscle performance with plasma antioxidant capacity were insignificant; 0.09 and 0.190.** (McLeay et al, 2012)

Antioxidant Properties of Berries: Review of Human Studies

Their Relevance in the Context of the European Food Safety Authority

Valeriya Krasovskaya
2012228, June 2012
Hogeschool van Amsterdam
Bacheloropleiding Voeding en Diëtetiek
http://kennisbank.hva.nl/document/478688

The following information was excerpted or modified from (Krasovskaya, 2012).
(Krasovskaya, 2012)

The Case of The Blueberry

The blueberry is a shrub belonging to the Heath (Ericaceae) family, whose other members are bilberry, cranberry, azalea, mountain laurel, and rhododendron. Blueberry color is purplish-blue. The berries' flavors can vary from mildly tart (wild berries) to sweet (cultivated species).

According to some, there are three varieties of blueberries: highbush (most commonly cultivated), lowbush (also referred to as "wild") and rabbiteye. Blueberries are found on the Euro-Asian, American and Australian continents.

Highbush varieties are found exclusively in North America.

Blueberries do not contain outstanding amounts of antioxidant vitamins; their in vitro antioxidant capacity has been attributed to the high concentration of phenolic compounds, particularly anthocyanins.

Latin names for blueberry sorts:

Vaccinium corymbosum L (Highbush)

Vaccinium angustifolium (Lowbush)

Vacciniumashei reade (Rabbiteye)

Vaccinium myrtillus L (Bilberry)

The United States supplies more than half of the global consumption of blueberries followed by Canada.

The state of Maine is the largest lowbush blueberry producer in the world.

Generally, the small-berried genotypes have much higher levels of anthocyanins than the large-berried genotypes.

The total antioxidant capacity of both highbush and lowbush blueberries species is about 3-fold higher than of strawberries or raspberries.

To date, blueberry is the most studied in clinical conditions among all berry types.

Health claims most commonly attributed to blueberry (however, they vary):

Improves vision

lowers blood sugar

rich in antioxidants

beneficial for intestinal health

The total oxygen radical absorbance capacity (ORAC) value of 11 anthocyanins (ACN) identified in blueberry is up to 12.83 mmol of TE/g fresh product and accounts for 56.3% of the total ORAC value. It basically means that **the ACN in blueberries are the major contributor to its antioxidant capacity**. (Zheng, Wang, 2010)

ACN from blueberry are sensitive to alkaline conditions (>7.0), high temperature (>80 °C) and direct strong light. Freezing does not influence significantly total anthocyanins content in blueberries, while dry berries, in contrast, have a lower ACN level than fresh ones. (Lohachoompol et al, 2004) (Wang et al, 2010)

In a study on cellular antioxidant activity of 25 common fruits wild blueberry was the champion in demonstrating antioxidant activity. Namely, **wild blueberry had the highest phenolic content, the highest ORAC score and the highest cellular antioxidant activity**. (Wolfe et al, 2008)

The study "Blueberry Supplementation Improves Memory in Older Adults" of Krikorian et al. was excluded from the review, as it did not contain any obvious links to antioxidant mechanisms.

In the last decennium some of the berry products, traditionally used in certain parts of the world, have appeared on market shelves of the other parts under the label **"superfoods"**. The efficient marketing policies, making use of selected scientific research, have resulted in rapidly increasing sales numbers.

The marketers largely stress antioxidant properties of berries. There is an outstanding number of research available on antioxidant activity of different berries. However, **most of the research is represented by *in vitro* experiments, followed by animal studies**.

Human research is still scarce and often operate with the markers which are not considered reliable enough to substantiate health claims.

The European Food Safety Authority (EFSA) is the body responsible for authorization of health claims within the European Union. The authorization of 222 out of 2758 health claims and their adoption by the European Commission on May 16 2012 has raised sound discussions within food industry. **None of the submitted berry claims have been authorized.**

Both consumers and trained nutritionists lack the accessible overview of the data available on the health benefits of the berries/their constituents.

So far, for none of the studied berries, including blueberries, is there a satisfactory (from the EFSA perspective) body of research available for substantiation of health claims related to antioxidant activities.

More human long-term well-designed studies should take place before any antioxidant-related claim can get the green light in the European Union.

More common to the US and European audiences berries such as blueberries and cherries are also being intensively promoted by institutions such as U.S. Highbush Blueberry Council and Cherry Marketing Institute correspondingly. Those institutions stimulate and collect the research on health benefits of the berries and make it available to the public. The available experimental data have led to a vast number of health claims ascribed to berries by the marketers, presenting them as **"cure all" products**.

A **free radical** (an EMOD or ROS) is readily formed when a covalent bond between entities is broken: basically, it is **by definition an atom or a group of atoms with at least one unpaired electron in the outermost shell**. An electron without a pair is unstable and can be highly reactive.

A free radical involving oxygen can be referred to as reactive oxygen species (ROS) or an electronically modified oxygen derivative (EMOD).

A free radical **accepts** an electron from a neighboring molecule, and thus a new free radical is formed in its place.

The newly formed radical again accepts an electron from another molecule, and a chain reaction can occur *in vitro*, which, if not intercepted by the antioxidative network, leads to oxidative damage.

ROS (EMODs) have the potential to damage vital biological systems and are incriminated to contribute to the aging process and to over a hundred of disease conditions. (Rolfes, Whitney, 2009) (Cao, Prior, 1998)

Halliwell & Gutteridge defined an antioxidant as 'any substance that, when present at low concentrations compared with that of an oxidizable substrate, significantly delays or inhibits oxidation of that substrate'. (Halliwell, Gutteridge, 1989)

RMH Note: The changed definition of the term "antioxidant" markedly expanded the wide spectrum of so-called antioxidants, including many other so-called antioxidants than just small electron donating molecules.

Polyphenols exhibit evident antioxidant properties as well. The exact mechanisms are being extensively studied and are not always clear yet.

Phytochemicals are bioactive non-nutrient plant compounds. **More than 10,000**

phytochemicals have been identified to date, but a large percentage still remains unknown. Phytochemicals are responsible for food's color, flavor, aroma, taste and other characteristics. In human body phytochemicals can mimic hormones, act as antioxidants and probably suppress development of diseases.

Polyphenols (previously called collectively Vitamin P) are plant secondary metabolites. They are physiologically essential for processes as plants' growth, pigmentation, lignification, pollination, allelopathy to name a few.

Several thousand polyphenols have been identified to date, and several hundred of them have been found in edible plants. The antioxidant characteristics of the polyphenols are due to the hydrogen of the phenoxyl groups that is prone to be donated to a radical, and by the ensuing structure that is chemically stabilized by resonance.

Flavonoids are a chemically defined class of polyphenols which have a basic structure as shown on the Figure2, and several subclasses of flavonoids are characterized by a substitution pattern in the B- and C-rings.

There have been identified approximately 8,000 individual flavonoids. Most of the flavonoids are present in plants with sugars attached (glycosides), although occasionally they are found as aglycones. Most of the research is concentrated on flavonoids with a common C6-C3-C6 structure consisting of 2 aromatic rings linked through an oxygenated heterocycle. The main subclasses include flavan-3-ols (catechin, epicatechin), flavanones (hesperetin), flavones (luteolin, apigenin), isoflavones(genistein), flavonols(quercetin, kaempferol, myricetin), and anthocyanidins.

The word anthocyanin originates from Greek anthos (flower) and kyanos (blue).

Anthocyanin is a conjugated anthocyanidin. It is the blue, red, blue-red, or purple water soluble pigment in berries, fruits, vegetables and leafs. It prevails in the skin of fruit and in buds and young shoots, and is an underlying pigment of chlorophyll in leaves, which becomes apparent as a purplish hue during late autumn.

Approximately 400 individual ACN have been identified to date. ACN contain a positively charged oxygen in the central group of the molecule. Chemically anthocyanins are subdivided into the sugar-free anthocyanidine aglycons and the anthocyanin glycosides. **The most widespread anthocyanin is cyanidin 3-glucoside**.

The greater the amount of ACN, the more intense the color of the plant. **Particularly dark purple berries (blueberry, black raspberry) are rich in anthocyanins.** ACN content in berries varies from 200 to 400 mg/100 g, increasing with the ripening process.

Average amount of ACN consumed throughout the world is reported from 12.5 mg to 225 mg of anthocyanins daily. The positively charged oxygen atom in the anthocyanin molecule makes it a more potent and distinct hydrogen donating antioxidant compared to other flavonoids.

Bioavailability presupposes "that a fraction of an ingested nutrient or compound that reaches the systemic circulation and the specific sites can exert its biological action."

The potential health benefits of berry polyphenols depend largely on their bioavailability.

From the meta study of Williamson et al. reviewing 93 articles **on the issue of bioavailability it can be concluded that the most well-absorbed polyphenols are gallic acid and isoflavones, followed by catechins, flavanones, and quercetin glucosides.** (Williamson, Manach, 3005) (Wu et al, 2002)

The least well-absorbed polyphenols are proanthocyanidins, catechins, and anthocyanins.

Authorized antioxidant claims ESFA has authorized claims on copper, manganese, riboflavin (Vitamin B2), selenium, vitamin C, vitamin E, and zinc with the wording contributes to the protection of cells from oxidative stress. All of these claims were authorized, because the EFSA concluded that the role of the reference vitamins and minerals as (indirect) components of the antioxidant defense system had been well established.

The only ESFA authorized of all the proposed claims on antioxidant activity of food/food constituents so far is the claim on polyphenols in olive oil, with the wording Contribute to the protection of blood lipids from oxidative stress.

In the last two decennia an impressive number of studies have been implemented on the potential health benefits of berries.

Most of the studies are in vitro experiments focusing on quantification of polyphenols, their metabolic pathways and effect on different biomarkers. The vast majority of this research hypothesizes that health benefits of the berries are due to their antioxidative capacities.

Numerous animal studies are also available. **There is still a lack of reliable human data.** Randomized controlled clinical trials are difficult to organize and are expensive.

Relevance of the studies in the context of EFSA

To date, 2012, there are eight human studies available on antioxidant properties of blueberries.

One of them, the study of Conception et. al, is a study on eating pattern and therefore is irrelevant in the scientific discourse. Trials of Wu et al. and Mazza et al. **are studies on bioavailability of blueberry ACN and therefore are only on the tertiary level of the EFSA hierarchy of scientific data.** (Wu et al, 2002)

Studies of Kay and Holub and Prior et al. measured changes in antioxidant status in plasma, **which is not directly related to any beneficial physiological effect in humans.** (Kay, Holub, 2002) (Prior et al, 2007)

Three other studies -- McAnulty et al., McAnulty et al., Wilms et al. operated with the markers which, if used alone, could not be considered sufficient for scientific substantiation from the EFSA's point of view. (McAnulty et al, 2005) (McAnulty et al, 2004) (Wilms et al, 2007)

Blueberry and EFSA

In total, eleven entries were indexed by the EFSA on blueberry/blueberry products. For the overview of the non-authorized claims please refer to the appendix Overview nonauthorized antioxidant activity related claims on berries/berry products. In summary, three of these claims have not been assessed, because the product was not sufficiently characterized.

For one another claim, the claimed effect was not sufficiently defined to be able to be assessed. For the remaining two claims, the claimed effect has not been substantiated, **"because no human studies which investigated the effects of the food(s)/food constituent(s) on reliable markers of oxidative damage to body cells or to molecules such as DNA, proteins and lipids were provided."**

The latter two claims were proposed for fresh blueberries and blueberry extracts and included the following wording, correspondingly: "Natural antioxidant, protect organism from oxidative damage, natural way to avoid risks caused by oxidation and peroxidation process" and "Natural berries contain plenty of natural antioxidants (polyphenolic compounds, Vitamin C and carotenoids) and fiber but only a small amount of energy and sodium. For this reason they are very suitable for a heart-friendly diet."

Withdrawn blueberry-related claims

The following blueberry-related claims have been withdrawn by the applicants:

- Claim nr. 3938: Vaccinium myrtillus (common name: blueberry, bilberry) – Astringent

- Claim nr. 2163: VitaBlue® Blueberry Extract 40% Total Phenolics – Excellent source of healthy fruit polyphenols known to help in the management of heart health

- Claim nr. 2162: VitaBlue® Wild Blueberry Extract – Excellent source of healthy fruit antioxidants. (EU register, 2012)

Two more blueberry-related claims (entry nr 2347 and 2050), which were categorized as "botanical substances", are still awaiting completion of the authorization process, together with other 2200 "botanical" claims.

It could be concluded that available human trials were low-scale and operated with the markers which, if used alone, could not be considered sufficient for scientific substantiation of health claims from the EFSA's point of view.

At this point, I have decided to include a brief discussion of the pomegranate, which I will expand upon in a subsequent book.

The Case of Pomegranate

The pomegranate (Latin name Punica granatum) is a fruit of a deciduous shrub belonging to Punicaceae family that grows up to 7 meters height. Inside the fruit, which on average is of an apple size, there are arils with 300-400 of edible seeds. The taste of the seeds varies depending on the sort and ripeness from sour to sweet with a hint of astringent taste deriving from the tannins.

Pomegranate juice is consumed world-wide, and is gaining more and more popularity. The highest antioxidant activity among pomegranate polyphenols was observed for punicalagin (the pomegranate ellagitannin).

Synonyms

Anardana, Dadim, Fruit of the Dead, Granada, Grenade, Roma, Shi Liu Gen Pi.

Interesting facts

The fruit is present in Persian and Greek mythologies, as well as in Hinduism and Chinese folklore, symbolizing life, marriage, fertility, prosperity and regeneration; **in Christianity its seeds are a symbol of individual worshipers gathered in one community of faith, while In Islam, the Quran indicates that pomegranates grow in the gardens of paradise.** (Ross, 2009)

Many scholars believe that the forbidden fruit that Eve seduced Adam with in the Garden of Eden was actually not an apple but a pomegranate.

The sales of pomegranate juice increased from $84,507 in 2001 to $66 million in 2005 in the United States. (Johanningsmeier, Harris, 2011)

Pomegranate and EFSA

There have been 12 applications made on pomegranate related health claims. The overview of the entries can be found in appendix Overview non-authorized antioxidant activity related claims on berries/berry products. Four of these entries were related to antioxidative properties of pomegranate/pomegranate juice. The EFSA Panel on Dietetic Products, Nutrition and Allergies (NDA) was asked to provide a scientific opinion on the pomegranate related health claims. The NDA issued its opinion in 2010. The active food constituents were defined as punicalagin/ellagic acid, and claimed effects were "antioxidative function", "antioxidant properties", and "antioxidants and immunity". The NDA assumed that the claimed effects related to the protection of lipids from oxidative damage caused by free radicals, which is a beneficial physiological effect.

In its opinion the NDA Panel summarized the provided human data for the proposed claims as follows:

A single arm, uncontrolled intervention study in 13 healthy male volunteers which assessed the effects of pomegranate juice consumption (50 mL per day containing 1.5 mmol total polyphenols) for two weeks on changes in the ex vivo activity of serum paraoxonase (an HDL associated esterase), in plasma lipid peroxides (AAPH induced spectrophotometric method), and in the oxidation lag time of low-density lipoproteins (LDL) ex vivo was provided. (Aviram et al., 2000)

A second single arm (Rosenblat et al., 2006), uncontrolled intervention study in 10 healthy subjects and 10 non-insulin dependent diabetes mellitus (NIDDM) patients under pharmacological treatment was provided with the consolidated list. (Rosenblat et al, 2006)

All subjects consumed 50 ml per day of pomegranate juice containing 1979 mg/l of tannins (1561 mg/L of punicalagin and 417 mg/l of hydrolysable tannins), 384 mg/l ofanthocyanins (delphinidin 3,5-diglucoside, cyanidin 3,5-diglucoside, delphinidin-3-glucoside, cyanidin 3-glucoside and pelargonidine 3-glucoside) and 121 mg/l of ellagic acid derivatives for three months. Serum concentrations of lipid peroxides, thiobarbituric acid reactive substances (TBARS), serum SH groups, serum paraoxonase 1 (PON1) activity, cellular peroxides and glutathione content in monocytes-derived macrophages (HMDM), and oxidized LDL uptake by HMDM were measured at the beginning and end of the intervention.

The NDA Panel considered that no conclusions could be drawn from these small and uncontrolled studies for the scientific substantiation of the claimed effect, and concluded that a cause and effect relationship was not established between the consumption of punicalagin/ellagic acid in pomegranate/pomegranate juice and the protection of lipids from oxidative damage.

Conclusions for Krasovskaya, 2012

Most studies report low flavonoids excretions, being particularly poor for anthocyanins, which are considered to play the major role in antioxidative mechanisms of berries (for instance in blueberries they are supposedly responsible for >50% of antioxidant activity). It could be therefore suggested that not all of the flavonoids' metabolites might have been identified yet, and that their bioavailability might be underestimated.

What needs to be noted is that **research teams worldwide have no consensus as how to assess metabolism of (berry) flavonoids and their impact on health.** Further (human) research is needed in order to design a reliable model for assessment of utilization of berries active compounds by the humans and their alleged benefits.

Of the five berries examined in this paper pomegranate shows to be the most promising in the sense, that the number of the human research available is the greatest for this fruit (although still not really impressive: 10 controlled clinical trials) and that some of the studies are long-term and/or operate with reliable markers (of oxidation).

As of 2012, the consumers should be aware that **sound claims of marketers on antioxidative properties of berries are not (sufficiently) substantiated from the scientific perspective.**

As berries are a safe, tasty and nutrient-dense, their consumption should be encouraged. (Krasovskaya, 2012)

I concur.

SECTION TWO

TOMATO ANTIOXIDANTS

(Lycopene)

Introduction

You have been led to believe that a healthy diet may **protect you against a variety of chronic health conditions**:

- Coronary heart disease

- Diabetes

- Osteoporosis

- High cholesterol

- High blood pressure

- Arthritis

- Certain types of cancer

So, why is it so hard to eat right?

Because there is no agreement as to what is "right."

And are tomatoes "super foods?"

Despite the adequate amount and variety of foods available, you might not be getting the best nutrition. In fact, the Centers for Disease Control and Prevention (CDC) notes that 38 percent of adults say they consume fruits less than once a day and nearly one quarter report not eating vegetables every day.

Additionally, more than 2 in 3 adults in the U.S. are overweight or obese.

Yet, many don't realize that they have a weight, diet and a health problem. So, they ignore health advice and warnings.

You might think that dietary changes made later in life will have little effect on your health. But changing and correcting dietary habits, exercising and losing weight in middle or even old age can significantly improve how you feel and can decrease your risk of chronic diseases.

Science based evidence is at the ground level of advances in the understanding and treatment of nutrition inadequacies, exercise deficiencies and weight control.

Lycopene is abundant in tomatoes, carrots, green peppers, and apricots.

Lycopene is concentrated by food processing and therefore may be found in high concentrations in foods such as processed tomato products (e.g., spaghetti sauce and tomato paste).

SUMMARIZED FACTOIDS ON TOMATO ANTIOXIDANTS

Lycopene factoid summary

- The landmark report of Block et al. in 1992 compiled the accumulated epidemiologic evidence associating fruit and vegetable intake with risk of cancers from an array of organs, concluding that diets rich in these components reduced the risk of many malignancies. (Block et al, 1992) **Yet, we are now a decade into the twenty first century and** we have no clear evidence that these recommendations are effective in reducing the cancer burden.

- The cultivated tomato has its origins as a wild small green fruit in the foothills of the Andes in the vicinity of present day Peru. (Peralta, Spooner, 2007)

- **Lycopene is not a necessary or essential nutrient**.

- Some have measured **carotenoid concentrations in human tissues, and lycopene is generally the highest carotenoid in individual tissues**. (Schmitz et al, 1991)

- **Lycopene is the most potent antioxidant for quenching singlet oxygen and scavenging free radicals**.

- **Lycopene is an excellent *in vitro* antioxidant, especially in quenching singlet oxygen, and may be the best dietary molecule in this regard**. (Di Mascio et al, 1989)

- **Cooking doesn't destroy lycopene**.

- **The optimum dosage for lycopene has not been established**.

- **Lycopene is about 3–5 times higher in concentration in the tomato skin compared to the pulp**. (Shi, Le Maguer, 2000)

- **Lycopene from tomato oleoresin or tomato juice (processed tomatoes) was better absorbed compared to lycopene from raw tomatoes**. (Bohm, Bitsch, 1999)

- **Use of lycopene appeared to reduce risk of preeclampsia.** Several other nutritional substances have shown promise for preventing preeclampsia in preliminary trials **only to fail when larger and more definitive studies were done**. (Sibai, 1998)

- The body uses some types of carotenoids (but **not lycopene**) to make vitamin A.

- Interest in lycopene did not really begin until the late 1980s when it was found that the antioxidant activity of lycopene was twice that of beta carotene.

Positive Studies

- Anti-proliferative effects of lycopene have been reported in several cancer cell lines **including those derived from prostate cancers and prostate epithelial cells**. (Chalabi et al, 2006) (Chalabi et al, 2007) (Tang et al, 2009) (Obermuller-Jevic et al, 2003) (Hasse et al, 2003) (Hwang et al, 2004) (Ivanov et al, 2007) (Sharoni et al, 2002) At this point in time, **it is clear that we have not established causality**.

- **A 2004 review that analyzed 21 observational studies (that is, not clinical trials) concluded that tomato products appear to have a weak protective effect against prostate cancer.** (American Cancer Society.org)

- **One animal study found that lycopene treatment reduced the growth of brain tumors. Another animal study showed that frequent intake of lycopene over a long period of time considerably suppressed breast tumor growth in mice.**

- **Lycopene supplements appeared to reduce the rapid growth of prostate cancer cells.** (American Cancer Society.org)

- Regarding yet another mouth condition, gingivitis (periodontal disease), **the results of a small double-blind trial suggest that lycopene can offer benefits when taken on its own, or when used to augment the effectiveness of standard care.** (Chandra et al, 2007)

- **Some of these studies report evidence for decreased prostate cancer risk with increased lycopene/tomato exposure.** (Comstock et al, 1991) (Le Marchand et al, 1991) (Schuman et al, 1982) (Goodman et al, 2003) (Wu et al, 2004) (Jian et al, 2005) (McCann et al, 2005) (Zhang et al, 2007) (Sanderson et al, 2004)

- The recent work of Mossine et al. provides an interesting twist to the concept that **freeze-dried tomato powder can inhibit prostate carcinogenesis.** The FruHis (a ketosamine)/lycopene combination significantly inhibited in vivo tumor formation by MAT-LyLu cells. (Mossine et al, 2008)

- A diet with **a high lycopene intake has the potential to improve cardiac event-free survival outcomes in heart failure (HF) patients.** (Biddle, et al, 2013)

Negative Studies

- **Carotenoids, while highly concentrated in many foods, are not well absorbed and rarely accumulate in high concentrations in blood and tissues.** (Lindshield, Erdman, 2006)

- **Unfortunately, the marketing of lycopene supplements and various related products, both by manufacturers and the popular press has misinformed the public with regards** to therapeutic outcomes and disease prevention. (Tan et al, 2010)

- It is not possible to recommend a specific dose of lycopene or foods containing lycopene in order to enhance health outcomes or prevent disease. (Moran et al, 2013)

- It seems unlikely that lycopene plays a meaningful a role as a fellow fat-soluble antioxidant. (Di Mascio et al, 1989)

- One human and six animal studies suggest that lycopene induces apoptosis of cancer cells, whereas one human study found no effect. (Kucuk et al, 2001)

- There is still no clearly proven clinical evidence supporting the use of lycopene in the prevention or treatment of prostate cancer, due to the only limited number of published randomized clinical trials and the varying quality of existing studies. (Holzapfel et al, 2013)

- In the trial by Talvas *et al.*, the PSA levels in the healthy men did not change after lycopene intervention. (Talvas et al, 2010)

- Pooling the results of the three trials revealed no statistically significant difference in the LDL lag time between the lycopene treatment group and the controlled group. (Jinyao et al, 2013)

- Until further research establishes significant health benefits for lycopene supplementation in humans, it should be concluded that the consumption of natural carotenoid-rich fruits and vegetables is preferential to purified lycopene supplementation. (Jinyao et al, 2013)

- Out of 2240 articles retrieved from databases and relevant bibliographies, 50 randomized controlled trials with 294,478 participants (156,663 in intervention groups and 137,815 in control groups) were included in the final analyses. In a fixed effect meta-analysis of the 50 trials, supplementation with vitamins and antioxidants was not associated with reductions in the risk of major cardiovascular events. (Myung et al, 2013) Among the subgroup meta-analyses by type of cardiovascular outcomes, *vitamin and antioxidant supplementation was associated with a marginally increased risk of angina pectoris.*

- There is no evidence to support the use of vitamin and antioxidant supplements for prevention of cardiovascular diseases. (Myung et al, 2013)

- Antioxidant vitamin supplementation has no effect on the incidence of major cardiovascular events, myocardial infarction, stroke, total death, cardiac death, revascularization, total CHD, angina and congestive heart failure. (Ye, Yuan, 2013)

- Although a number of strategies have been aimed at to ameliorate lethal reperfusion injury, up to date the beneficial effects in clinical settings have been disappointing [for antioxidant vitamins]. (Rodrigo et al, 2013)

- The intake of isolated lycopene does not protect from the development of prostate cancer (PCA). (Ellinger et al, 2009)

- Imaida et al. reported no significant effects of lycopene supplementation against rat prostate carcinogenesis. (Imaida et al, 2001)

- Lycopene can block the cancer killing ability of chemo and radiation therapy. Lycopene as an antioxidant scavenged reactive oxygen substances, prevented apoptosis, maintained normal function in Sertoli cells and helped to provide physical and metabolic support for sperm production, thereby treating infertility in men. (Krishnamoorthy et al, 2013)

- We did not detect significant individual genes associated with dietary intake and supplementation of lycopene and fish oil (micronutrients may modify the risk or delay progression of prostate cancer). (Magbanua et al, 2011)

- The bioactive compounds in garlic and/or tomato administered for a short period did not prevent or reduce the development of experimental Ehrlich ascites tumors in BALB/c mice. (Bom et al, 2014)

- Two studies from 2007, one of about 1,500 men and the second of more than 28,000 men, found no difference in blood lycopene levels between those in whom prostate cancer later developed and those in whom it did not. (American Cancer Society.org)

- There has been a human study that assigned men at high risk for prostate cancer to take an ordinary multivitamin either with or without a lycopene supplement. This study found no difference in prostate-specific antigen (**PSA, a marker of prostate cancer) levels between the 2 groups.** (American Cancer Society.org)

- **The rats that received tomato powder had much lower cancer risk, whereas the rats receiving lycopene supplements did not differ significantly from the group that received no special supplements.** (American Cancer Society.org)

- **A more recent study with men whose prostate cancer had stopped responding to hormone therapy found that lycopene did not have a significant effect.** (American Cancer Society.org)

- **One short-term study from 2006 reported that lycopene supplements were safe, but that they did not lower the levels of prostate-specific antigen (PSA, a marker of prostate cancer) in men with prostate cancer that had come back.** (American Cancer Society.org)

- Results of studies have been **inconsistent** regarding the effects of lycopene and exercise-induced asthma. (Falk et al, 2995) (Neuman et al, 2000)

- **One observational study failed to find that high consumption of lycopene reduced risk of developing diabetes.** (Wang et al, 2006)

- In the **May 2007 issue of Cancer Epidemiology, Biomarkers & Prevention**, researchers based at the National Cancer Institute and Fred Hutchinson Cancer Research Center report that **lycopene, an antioxidant predominately found in tomatoes, does not effectively prevent prostate cancer.** In fact, *the researchers noted an association between beta-carotene, an antioxidant related to lycopene, and an increased risk for aggressive prostate cancer.* Study data were derived from over **28,000 men enrolled in the Prostate, Lung, Colorectal, and Ovarian (PLCO) Cancer Screening Trial**, an ongoing, **randomized National Cancer Institute trial** to evaluate cancer screening methods and to investigate early markers of cancer.

- In a 2006 study, **Ulrike Peters, Ph.D., M.P.H., of the Fred Hutchinson Cancer Research Center and her colleagues looked at the dietary intake of more than 25 tomato-based foods, also using data from the PLCO trial, and found no**

overall association between lycopene intake and prostate cancer.

- They found no significant difference between those who had prostate cancer and those who did not in relation to the concentration of lycopene in their bloodstream. "Our results do not offer support for the benefits of lycopene against prostate cancer," Peters said. **Most surprisingly, says Peters, was the relationship between increased risk of aggressive prostate cancer – defined as disease that has spread beyond the prostate – and beta-carotene, another antioxidant found in many vegetables and commonly used as a dietary supplement**.

- According to a review conducted by the U.S. Food and Drug Administration (FDA), **there is "no credible evidence" that lycopene reduces the risk of cancers such as prostate cancer, and "very limited evidence" that tomato consumption reduces risk**. The review was published in the *Journal of the National Cancer Institute*.

- In response to groups who wanted to make claims about the cancer benefits of lycopene or tomatoes, in 2007, **the FDA conducted a review of the available scientific evidence**. The main conclusions of the review were the following:

- **There is no credible evidence that lycopene reduces the risk of prostate, lung, colorectal, gastric, breast, ovarian, endometrial, or pancreatic cancer.**

- **There is no credible evidence that tomato consumption reduces the risk of lung, colorectal, breast, cervical, or endometrial cancer.**

- **There is very limited evidence that tomato consumption reduces the risk of prostate, ovarian, gastric, and pancreatic cancer.**

(Kavanaugh et al, 2007)

In an accompanying editorial, Dr. Edward Giovannucci addressed possible reasons for the inconsistent results of previous studies. (Giovannucci, 2007)

- **Developing laboratory research suggests lycopene might worsen established prostate cancer by increasing the spread of cancer without having any effect on cancer cell growth.**

- **Overall, neither lycopene nor curcumin can consistently prevent rat prostate carcinogenesis.** (Imaida et al, 2001)

- **Some studies failed to demonstrate anticancer efficacy of lycopene in the liver, colon, urinary bladder and lung.** (Kim et al, 1997) (Okajima et al, 1997) (Hect et al, 1999) (Cohen et al, 1999)

- **Our study did not find a blood pressure lowering effect of dark chocolate or tomato extract in a prehypertensive population.** Practicability of chocolate as a long-term treatment option may be limited. (Reid et al, 2009)

- **Blood pressure, arterial stiffness, lipids and hsCRP levels were unchanged for lycopene vs. placebo treatment groups in the CVD arm as well as the HV arm. Lycopene supplementation improves endothelial function in CVD patients on optimal secondary prevention, but not in healthy volunteers (HVs).** (Gajendragadkar et al, 2014)

- **Until now, human intervention studies mostly failed to show any CVD prevention. There are a lot of investigations needed in the future to give reliable results to establish these CVD-preventive effects.** (Bohm, 2012)

- **In a randomized controlled trial, lycopene supplementation in moderately overweight, disease-free, middle aged adults (an appropriate target population for lycopene supplementation in clinical practice) showed no significant changes in markers of cardiovascular disease. These findings do not justify potential health claims that lycopene supplementation has a cardioprotective effect.** (Thies et al, 2012)

- **There is limited support for the *in vivo* antioxidant function for lycopene. Moreover, tissue levels of lycopene appear to be too low to play a meaningful antioxidant role.** We conclude that **there is an overall shortage of supportive evidence for the "antioxidant hypothesis" as lycopene's major in vivo mechanism of action.** Our laboratory has postulated that metabolic products of lycopene, **the lycopenoids, may be responsible for some of lycopene's reported bioactivity.** (Erdman, Ford, Lindshield, 2008)

- Whereas, **some lycopene studies show little to no effect.** (Hayes et al, 1999) (Sonada et al, 2004) (Bosetti et al, 2004) (Kirsh et al, 2006) (Chang et al, 2005) (Peters et al, 2007) (Key et al, 2007) (Pourmand et al, 2007)

Prof Randolph M Howes MD,PhD

Lycopene according to WebMD

WebMD website: http://www.webmd.com/vitamins-supplements/ingre-dientmono-554-lycopene.aspx?activeingredientid=554&activeingredientname=lycopene

Lycopene is a naturally occurring chemical that gives fruits and vegetables a red color. It is one of a number of pigments called carotenoids.

Lycopene is found in watermelons, pink grapefruits, apricots, and pink guavas. It is found in particularly high amounts in tomatoes and tomato products.

In North America, 85% of dietary lycopene comes from tomato products such as tomato juice or paste. One cup (240 mL) of tomato juice provides about 23 mg of lycopene.

Processing raw tomatoes using heat (in the making of tomato juice, tomato paste or ketchup, for example) actually changes the lycopene in the raw product into a form that is easier for the body to use. The lycopene in supplements is about as easy for the body to use as lycopene found in food.

People take lycopene for preventing heart disease, "hardening of the arteries" (atherosclerosis); and cancer of the prostate, breast, lung, bladder, ovaries, colon, and pancreas. Lycopene is also used for treating human papilloma virus (HPV) infection, which is a major cause of uterine cancer. Some people also use lycopene for cataracts and asthma.

How does it work?

Lycopene is a powerful antioxidant that **allegedly may help** protect cells from damage. This is why there is a lot of research interest in lycopene's role in preventing cancer.

Other names for lycopene: All-trans lycopene, Cis-lycopene, Licopeno, Psi-Pse carotene.

Tomato and prostate cancer prevention: what have we learned?

The following has been excerpted or modified from: (Tan et al, 2010)

96

Evidence derived from a vast array of laboratory studies and epidemiological investigations have implicated diets rich in fruits and vegetables with a reduced risk of certain cancers. However, these approaches cannot demonstrate causal relationships and there is a paucity of randomized, controlled trials due to the difficulties involved with executing studies of food and behavioral change.

At this point in time, there are no chemopreventive strategies that are standard of care in medical practice. This review describes an alternative approach focusing upon development of tomato-based food products for human clinical trials targeting cancer prevention and as an adjunct to therapy. Tomatoes are a source of bioactive phytochemicals and are widely consumed.

Cancer epidemiology emerged as a rapidly growing discipline and it was soon realized that migrant populations often developed cancer risk profiles of the host nation in conjunction with adoption of new cultural and lifestyle patterns, strongly implicating environmental influences as opposed to inherited genetics as the primary driver of cancer risk.

One theme that emerged and has been adopted for public health recommendations is the potential for diets rich in fruits and vegetables to inhibit various types of cancer.

The landmark report of Block et al. in 1992 compiled the accumulated epidemiologic evidence associating fruit and vegetable intake with risk of cancers from an array of organs, concluding that diets rich in these components reduced the risk of many malignancies. (Block et al, 1992)

The 1997 report of the AICR/WCRF, which was updated in 2007, was the most thorough review of diet and cancer risk ever undertaken, and also concluded that **a plant-based diet was the foundation for a cancer prevention dietary pattern.** (WCRF, 1997)

Yet, we are now a decade into the twenty first century and **we have no clear evidence that these recommendations are effective in reducing the cancer burden.**

Ideally, the documentation of bioactive components in the food of interest that demonstrate anticancer activity using a combination of preclinical in vitro and in vivo approaches and characterization of biomarkers of exposure and of efficacy that can be applied to human translational studies, are necessary for moving forward with definitive prevention trials. Initial human studies (phase I and II) focus upon defining optimal dosages that provide excellent compliance, with safety, and impact bio-markers of activity. (MacDonald et al, 2009)

Definitive phase III trials must also consider the population to target, which is likely driven by funding available.

In this review, the focus is on developing novel tomato (Solanum lycopersicum) products for cancer prevention studies, with a particular emphasis upon prostate cancer.

Tomato domestication and horticulture

The present-day tomato does not have a long history of human consumption. Considerable genetic evidence suggests that **the cultivated tomato has its origins as a wild small green fruit in the foothills of the Andes in the vicinity of present day Peru**. (Peralta, Spooner, 2007)

One species, a yellow variety the size of current cherry tomatoes, was domesticated, cultivated, and consumed by the Aztecs of Central America, which they called xitomatl, starting around 700 AD. Early in the 15th century, tomato seeds were first introduced to Europe and other parts of the globe by the Spanish, likely from the Central American cultivars after colonization. (Smith et al, 2001) (Smith AF, Peralta IE, Spooner DM. Early history, culture, and cookery. Vol. 5. University of Illinois Press; 2001)

Records identifying tomato use in Europe were documented in 1544 in Italy but **they were considered toxic** and therefore predominantly used for ornamental purposes while gradually integrating into European cuisine over the next two centuries. (Smith et al, 2001)

Throughout the 1800s, toxicity concerns were dispelled and consumption increased in many areas of the world. Tomato production soared by the 1920s with the application of safe mass canning that built upon the development of mechanized peeling, juice extraction, and sterilization techniques.

With increasing demand and knowledge derived from horticultural genetics, more desirable features were selected for varietal improvement to improve appearance, size, and quality of fruit. Over recent decades, selection of strains to enhance disease resistance, improve mechanical harvesting, facilitate processing to various products, and impact ripening and transportation has promoted the economic value of tomatoes.

Current consumer interest in potential health benefits, tomato quality and organic farming, with continued anxiety over genetic manipulation, has created many avenues for the further development of tomatoes with diverse characteristics to target various stakeholders, including those on both the production and consumption sides.

Tomato production and consumption

Tomatoes are a popular food item and a generally acceptable addition to the diet of those at risk for cancer. The global annual production of tomatoes is nearly 130 Mt (1 Mt=10^6 t) and the USA currently ranks second in production.

By weight, the tomato ranks third in global production of fruits and vegetables behind potatoes and sweet potatoes. In the USA, the tomato ranks fifth in crop production behind potatoes, lettuce, onions, and watermelon.

The annual per capita consumption in the USA averages approximately 20 lb of fresh tomatoes and 70 lb of processed tomatoes divided among sauces (35%), followed by paste (18%), canned whole tomato products (17%), and catsup and juice (each about 15%).

Bioactive phytochemicals in tomatoes

The emergence of epidemiological studies suggesting health benefits of tomatoes immediately led to speculation regarding the potential bioactive components that may mediate the putative benefits, with a major focus upon carotenoids.

Lycopene, the carotenoid providing the red color to tomatoes, was an easy target as the United States Department of Agriculture (USDA) had extensive food analysis data defining carotenoid content of foods due to the importance of carotenoids (β-carotene and other provitamin A carotenoids) in providing vitamin A in the diet. The rapid commercialization of lycopene supplements and tomato extracts marketed to consumers soon followed.

However, with time, several lines of evidence indicated that **a reductionist approach, focusing only upon lycopene, may be too simplistic.** Indeed, **our studies of experimental prostate cancer in rodent models indicated that tomato powder was more effective than lycopene in the inhibition of carcinogenesis.** (Boileau et al, 2003) (Canene-Adams et al, 2007)

Tomatoes are cholesterol-free and low in fat and calories, thus often incorporated into a healthy dietary pattern. Tomatoes are typically 5–10% dry matter, nearly half of which is reducing sugars and about 10% organic acids, primarily citrate and malate.

Non-provitamin A carotenoids such as lycopene, phytoene, and phytofluene are the focus of significant attention. An array of polyphenols are also present, primarily as flavonoids, with the USDA nutrient bank reporting that flavanones (e.g., naringenin), flavones (e.g., apigenin and luteolin), and flavonols (e.g., kaempferol, myricetin, quercetin) are the major components.

The major effort thus far has focused upon the carotenoids and polyphenols as the active anticancer components.

Epidemiology of tomato intake, lycopene exposure and prostate cancer

The hypothesis that diets rich in tomatoes may have a role in prostate cancer prevention was driven primarily by epidemiological investigations. The fact that the USDA also had a database for carotenoid content of foods allowed epidemiologists to link estimated intakes of tomato products with the average carotenoid content to obtain an estimate of lycopene exposure.

Thus, the focus of attention was immediately upon lycopene, as opposed to other phytochemicals, and was further facilitated by the ability to measure serum lycopene concentrations as a biomarker of exposure by HPLC for additional epidemiologic investigations.

The landmark publication by Giovannucci et al. is illustrative of the important prospective cohort studies that support the tomato–prostate cancer hypothesis. The report is derived from the prospective Health Professional's Follow-up Study, a cohort of over 50,000 American men that has been monitored since 1984. (Giovannucci et al, 1995)

Among the dozens of vegetables and fruits or related products examined, **the authors reported a significantly lower prostate cancer risk for tomato sauce, tomatoes, and pizza**. Using the USDA database for carotenoid content of foods, the authors examined the relationship of carotenoids to risk. They observed no relationship between β-carotene, α-carotene, lutein, and β-crypotoxanthin and prostate cancer; only lycopene intake was associated with a lower risk.

The combined intake of tomatoes, tomato sauce, tomato juice, and pizza (accounting for 82% of lycopene intake) was inversely associated with risk of prostate cancer and locally advanced or metastatic prostate cancers.

The Physician's Health Study is the largest plasma-based study to date. Gann et al. showed that plasma lycopene level was significantly lower in all prostate cancer cases and in aggressive phenotype. Similarly, **other studies, but not all, generally confirmed the inverse associations between elevated blood lycopene level and diminished prostate cancer risk.** (Lu et al, 2001) (Wu, Erdman, Schwartz et al, 2004)

The accurate assessment of dietary intake is always a concern, although the current food-frequency questionnaires have been continually improved, error both in the quantity of specific foods consumed and the frequency adds to the imprecision of assessing relationships between tomato products and prostate cancer risk.

The estimation of lycopene intake from the food frequency questionnaire is even more problematic, as the variability of lycopene content in foods can be quite significant based upon the source of tomatoes, ripeness, processing, and cooking.

Case–control studies are also plagued by reporting bias as cases typically will recall dietary patterns differently than when assessed prior to diagnosis. (Giovannucci, 1999) (Giovannucci, 2005)

Thus, when we consider these issues in total, it is indeed remarkable that a trend toward a protective effect of tomatoes has emerged when the data is examined as a whole.

Although continued efforts to elucidate relationships between tomato exposure and prostate cancer risk are worthy to consider, the focus should be on prospective studies of sufficient statistical power and precision in the assessment of diet and cancer outcomes.

Nutritional epidemiology provided estimated exposure to lycopene and suggested correlations with reduced risk. Thus, the hypothesis that lycopene could mediate the anti-prostate cancer activity of tomato intake emerged rapidly and was particularly supported by the food and supplement industry. **If a relationship truly exists, biological plausibility must be established by correlative scientific data.**

Thus, **the human prostate contains lycopene and other dietary carotenoids**, supporting the hypothesis that tomato-derived carotenoids may directly impact the prostate. Interestingly, we continue to speculate on the role of cis-isomers and their potential to impact biology.

Intervention studies of tomatoes or lycopene and prostate cancer

There are no long-term cancer prevention studies of tomatoes or lycopene for prostate cancer prevention. However, intervention studies have provided some provocative data. **Serum lycopene concentrations can change quickly with alterations in the daily intake of tomato products.**

Allen et al. reported changes in plasma lycopene concentrations in healthy adults consuming standard daily servings of processed tomato products: tomato sauce (21 mg lycopene per serving), soup (12 mg lycopene per serving), or juice (17 mg lycopene per serving) for 4 weeks. Total plasma lycopene concentrations during a 2-week washout period. **Following intervention, plasma lycopene concentrations increased significantly for those consuming sauce, soup, and juice to 2.08 µM, respectively.** (Allen et al, 2003)

Bowen et al. provided pre-prostatectomy patients with 3 weeks of a tomato sauce-based pasta meal providing 30 mg of lycopene per day. **After the dietary intervention, serum and prostate lycopene concentrations were statistically significantly increased, from 0.6 and from 0.28 µmol/g, respectively.** (Bowen et al, 2002)

These examples illustrate that **changing the daily intake of tomato products or lycopene oleoresin will significantly impact serum and prostate tissue lycopene concentrations over a relatively short period of a few weeks.**

In addition, the studies provide provocative correlative data suggesting the potential to impact PSA and other markers of activity, **yet all studies thus far reported are very limited in statistical power and these findings must be considered with caution.**

Imaida et al. reported no significant effects of lycopene supplementation against rat prostate carcinogenesis. (Imaida et al, 2001)

Studies have investigated the combined effects of lycopene, vitamin E, and selenium, yet the rodent studies cannot differentiate the individual impact of lycopene. A study in a transplantable model of prostate tumorigenesis showed that **tomato powder was more effective than lycopene for the inhibition of tumor growth**. (Canene-Adams et al, 2007)

Boileau et al. compared a control diet to those fed diets containing tomato powder or lycopene in a rat model with prostate cancer induced by testosterone and N-nitroso-N-methylurea. The control group experienced the greatest risk of prostate cancer, with tomato powder fed rats showing the lowest risk, with lycopene-fed rats experiencing an intermediate risk. In this study, plasma lycopene concentrations were similar in both tomato powder and lycopene-fed animals although the lycopene content in the tomato powder diet was approximately ten times lower than the lycopene beadlet diet. (Boileau et al, 2003)

Thus illustrating, absorption of lycopene in the rats can be saturated. In addition, it is clear **that absorption of lycopene by rats and mice is less efficient than in humans,** a fact that should be considered in the design of studies.

The recent work of Mossine et al. provides an interesting twist to the concept that **freeze-dried tomato powder can inhibit prostate carcinogenesis**. The FruHis (a ketosamine)/lycopene combination significantly inhibited in vivo tumor formation by MAT-LyLu cells. (Mossine et al, 2008)

Thus, **FruHis or other ketosamines may be non-carotenoid components of tomato products that could inhibit prostate carcinogenesis**.

Overall, the studies in rodent models are supportive of a protective effect of tomato products on prostate carcinogenesis and tumorigenesis, with a less potent, but detectable impact of pure lycopene. Thus, **lycopene is likely one component, but not the only component of tomatoes that impact prostate cancer risk.**

Tomatoes are a rich source of carotenoids, particularly lycopene that provides the familiar red color of tomato. Although up to 20 different carotenoids have been detected in tomatoes, **lycopene will typically account for 70–90% of carotenoids present**, approximately 3–5 mg/100g of raw fruit, which is defined by genetics, environmental factors, and state of ripening.

Lycopene is about 3–5 times higher in concentration in the tomato skin compared to the pulp. (Shi, Le Maguer, 2000)

The impact, if any, of a low-dose exposure to the carotenoid array found in tomatoes for cancer prevention, as opposed to pharmacologic approaches with lycopene alone, is not well understood. **It remains a viable hypothesis, but not proven, that the pattern of carotenoids may underlie the greater benefits of tomato products compared to lycopene**.

Lycopene absorption and bioavailability

Carotenoid absorption is highly variable, yet we are elucidating many factors that impact the process. Isomerization of lycopene impacts absorption efficiency. Cis-isomers of lycopene are produced during processing and cooking of tomato products, in addition, some isomerization may occur in the gastrointestinal tract, especially in the environment of the stomach.

Studies with lymph-cannulated ferrets demonstrated that a lycopene dose that contained <10% cis-lycopene, lead to higher concentrations of cis-isomers in the small intestinal mucosal cells (58%), mesenteric lymph (77%), serum (52%), and tissues (47–58%), primarily the 5-cis-isomer.

Lycopene from tomato oleoresin or tomato juice (processed tomatoes) was better absorbed compared to lycopene from raw tomatoes. (Bohm, Bitsch, 1999)

Age may be another factor impacting lycopene absorption. The bioavailability of lycopene was less in those 60–75 years of age compared to those 20–35.

Mechanisms of Lycopene and tomatoes on prostate cancer

Although epidemiology is suggestive and rodent models are supportive of the anti-prostate cancer effects of tomatoes and lycopene, the underlying mechanisms remain very speculative.

Lycopene is hypothesized to protect critical biomolecules such as DNA, protein, and lipids from free radical damage. On the contrary, **in vivo evidence for this activity is difficult to document**.

Consumption of tomato products decreased DNA damage, LDL oxidation, production of lipid peroxide, and oxidative stress in lymphocytes. Two studies also demonstrated no beneficial effects from lycopene supplements despite higher lycopene levels compared with tomato product supplementation.

Anti-proliferative effects of lycopene have been reported in several cancer cell lines **including those derived from prostate cancers and prostate epithelial cells**. (Chalabi, Delort et al, 2006) (Chalabi et al, 2007) (Tang et al, 2009) (Obermuller-Jevic et al, 2003) (Hasse et al, 2003) (Hwang et al, 2004) (Ivanov et al, 2007) (Sharoni et al, 2002)

At this time, 2010, a role for lycopene or other tomato phytochemicals in epigenetic regulation within the prostate and its impact on carcinogenesis is speculative.

At this point in time, **it is clear that we have not established causality**, and this issue has been previously addressed. The chemical instability of lycopene and other tomato-derived carotenoids requires that investigators take special precautions to insure quality and informative data. (Miller et al, 2002)

The concept that we can manipulate the tomato and create novel tomato-based food products, also known as functional foods that are specifically designed to target prostate carcinogenesis is very attractive, but with potential for harm.

Conclusions

The possibility that tomato products have anti-prostate cancer properties remains a viable hypothesis. **It is very clear that causality has not been established** and that significant amounts of additional research are necessary to solidify such a relationship.

Unfortunately, the marketing of lycopene supplements and various related products, both by manufacturers and the popular press has misinformed the public with regards to therapeutic outcomes and disease prevention. (Tan et al, 2010)

Interactions of lycopene on dietary and genetic factors

The following was excerpted or modified from: (Moran et al, 2013)

Intake of lycopene, a red, **tetraterpene carotenoid** found in tomatoes is epidemiologically associated with a decreased risk of chronic disease processes, and lycopene has demonstrated bioactivity in numerous *in vitro* and animal models. However, our understanding of absorption, tissue distribution, and biological impact in humans remains very limited. Lycopene absorption is strongly impacted by dietary composition, especially the amount of fat.

Lycopene is not uniformly distributed among tissues, with adipose, liver, and blood being the major body pools, while the testes, adrenals, and liver have the greatest concentrations compared to other organs.

Lycopene is a bioactive carotenoid found in tomatoes, watermelon, pink grapefruit, guava and several other red fruits. In the United States, men and women consume an average of 6.8 and 4.6 mg of lycopene/d, respectively.

The majority of dietary lycopene comes from tomatoes, thus plasma lycopene concentration is a robust biomarker of tomato intake.

Variations in host genes and nutrient status that influence body lycopene pools and bioactivity are just beginning to be elucidated.

Interest in the relationship of dietary lycopene to cancer risk began with associations between estimated intake of tomato products and risk, with approximate lycopene exposure being defined based upon an average concentration in tomato-containing food products. While this approach is fraught with challenges and assumptions, due to imprecision of dietary assessment tools over the life span and remarkable heterogeneity of lycopene content within specific tomato-based foods, many epidemiologic studies have reported a protective relationship, while as expected, many of limited statistical power fail to detect any relationship.

Recent reviews illustrate the current status of the literature with an emphasis on prostate and breast cancer. (Eliassen et al, 2012) (Wei, Giovannucci, 2012) (Etminan et al, 2004)

A better understanding of the absorption, distribution, metabolism, and excretion of lycopene provides an enhanced ability to interpret epidemiologic findings, plan physiologically-relevant animal and in vitromechanistic investigations, and to design interventions for clinical evaluation.

One important question concerns the half-life of lycopene in the body. Plasma lycopene half-life can provide insight into how frequently lycopene should be consumed in order to maintain a desired plasma concentration. **In one study in which 20 mg of lycopene from tomato soup or from synthetic lycopene tablets was consumed for 8 sequential days, plasma lycopene half-life was found to be 6.4 and 5.6 d, respectively.** (Cohn et al, 2004)

Differences in half-lives for lycopene geometrical isomers are likely due to a number of factors including the higher bioavailability of cis versus trans, endogenous isomerization, which may or may not be enzymatic, and greater thermodynamic stability of cis at elevated temperatures.

Lycopene concentrations in cancer tissue

The development of a malignancy within a tissue is associated with a change in the structure of the microenvironment and cellular metabolism, thus carotenoid uptake and biological impact may be different between a cancer and the adjacent "normal" tissue.

Prostate lycopene concentrations in tissue collected by prostatectomy from men with localized prostate cancer [23] differed significantly between cancerous and normal prostate tissues.

The effect of prostate cancer on lycopene accumulation in the prostate was examined in a randomized, double-blinded, placebo-controlled supplementation trial. Men with either prostate cancer or benign prostatic hyperplasia were treated for 3-wk with placebo or lycopene (30 mg lycopene/day as tomato extract supplement). While the cancerous vs. benign tissue lycopene concentrations were not statistically compared in the original publication, they were numerically presented for the placebo-control group as 0.52 ± 0.66 vs. 0.39 ± 0.42 nmol/g, for prostate cancer and benign prostatic hyperplasia (BPH) respectively and for the tomato extract-fed group as 0.71 ± 0.60 vs. 0.46 ± 0.43 nmol/g, in tissues from subjects with prostate cancer vs. BPH, respectively. (van Breeman et al, 2011)

Cancerous cells are typically more metabolically active than their non-cancerous counterparts. Perhaps an increased demand for preformed cholesterol by prostate tumors stimulates lipoprotein uptake, resulting in elevated lycopene co-transport into cancerous prostate tissue. (Twiddy et al, 2012)

Lycopene is generally understood to be distributed in the same manner as cholesterol, thus it may be hypothesized that lycopene is deposited extensively in cancerous prostate tissues as a result of perturbed cholesterol and lipoprotein homeostasis.

Though the cellular uptake and efflux of lycopene and its metabolites is still poorly understood, it is known that prostate cancers have elevated levels of cholesterol in the epithelial cells.

At this point in time, it is premature to make any conclusions regarding lycopene concentrations in cancer compared to nonmalignant counterparts.

Lycopene bioavailability in the proximal intestine is understood to be influenced by food processing and cooking, meal composition, mastication, and the isomeric configurations of lycopene.

Absorption and lycopene plasma concentrations are then influenced by the ability of transporters on absorptive intestinal cells to facilitate lycopene uptake and basolateral efflux from the enterocyte, an individual's lipid metabolic profile, the uptake and efflux transporters present on different cell types, and the activity of putative lycopene metabolizing enzymes.

Lycopene is a very lipophilic molecule, and therefore to be absorbed from a food it must be solubilized, first by emulsification in the gastric contents, then incorporation into mixed micelles in the duodenum as facilitated by bile acid surfactants and lipases. Co-consumed dietary fat is important, if not essential, for effectively solubilizing lycopene, stimulating the excretion of bile acids, and providing lipids to form the micelles.

In fasting plasma, lycopene is found primarily in LDL (76%), followed by HDL (17%) and VLDL (7%), thus it is plausible that genetic factors impacting lipoprotein metabolism are likely to impact lycopene plasma pharmacokinetics and tissue distribution. In fact, plasma cholesterol levels were significantly associated with plasma lycopene levels (P= 0.0001) and in a stepwise regression analysis, accounted for 14% of the variability in plasma lycopene in a study population (n = 111). Dietary lycopene, plasma triglycerides, and dietary vitamin C were also significantly correlated with plasma lycopene levels in this population. (Mayne et al, 1999)

The subcellular localization of lycopene in cells may also impact biological activity. In cultured prostate cancer cells (LNCaP, DU145, and PC-3), LNCaP cells accumulated the greatest amount of lycopene from the media, and the majority of this lycopene is found in the nuclear membranes (55%), followed by the nuclear matrix (26%), and microsomal fractions (19%), with lycopene being undetectable in the cytosol.

Summary

Studies from the epidemiological literature and a growing number of human clinical studies, coupled with accumulating evidence from the laboratory support the hypothesis that lycopene may have biological activity in humans and impact health or disease risk. **Yet, definitive causal**

relationships are very uncertain, and it is not possible to recommend a specific dose of lycopene or foods containing lycopene in order to enhance health outcomes or prevent disease.

Studies in humans suggest that lycopene exposure, absorption, metabolism, and bioactivity is quite complex. Many genes may impact lycopene absorption and metabolism and human variation in expression of these genes, due to regulatory factors or inherited polymorphisms, is only beginning to be understood.

Highlights

- There is wide tissue and plasma lycopene variability in response to dietary consumption.

- Dietary factors include fat amount and type, food matrix, and geometric isomeric configuration.

- Genetic factors may be lipid transporters, lipoproteins, and carotenoid cleavage enzymes.

- Most intact lycopene is found in adipose tissue, liver, and serum.

- Lycopene products include epoxides, alcohols, aldehydes, carboxylic acids, and carbon dioxide.

(Moran et al, 2013)

American Cancer Society. org website: Lycopene

http://www.cancer.org/treatment/treatmentsandsideeffects/complementaryandalternativemedicine/dietandnutrition/lycopene

It is one of the major carotenoids in the diet of North Americans and Europeans.

Carotenoids are pigments that give yellow, red, and orange vegetables and fruits their colors. The body uses some types of carotenoids, such as beta carotene (but **not lycopene**) to make vitamin A.

Eating lycopene-rich vegetables and fruits together with a small amount of oil or fat (for example, salad oil or cheese on pizza) increases the amount of lycopene absorbed by the intestines. Lycopene is also available in soft-gel capsule and liquid supplements.

The examination of the role of carotenoids, specifically beta carotene, in preventing cancer began in the 1920s. However, interest in lycopene did not really begin until the late 1980s when it was found that **the antioxidant activity of lycopene was twice that of beta carotene.**

What is lycopene's role?

Studies that look at large groups of people (observational studies) in many countries have shown that **the risk for some types of cancer is lower in people who have higher levels of lycopene in their blood**.

Studies suggest that diets rich in tomatoes may account for this reduction in risk. (Etminan et al, 2004) (Giovannucci, 2005)

Evidence is strongest for lycopene's protective effect against cancer of the lung, stomach, and prostate. It may also help to protect against cancer of the cervix, breast, mouth, pancreas, esophagus, and colon and rectum.

Some population studies have found that a diet high in lycopene from tomato-based foods was linked with a lower risk of prostate cancer. **Other studies, however, found no link between tomato products or other lycopene-rich foods and prostate cancer**.

A recent study suggested that variation in a particular gene (known as XRCC1) that helps repair damaged DNA influences whether lycopene intake will affect a man's prostate cancer risk. (Goodman et al, 2006)

A 2004 review that analyzed 21 observational studies (that is, not clinical trials) concluded that tomato products appear to have a weak protective effect against prostate cancer. This review did not include lycopene supplements, only tomato and tomato-based foods. Some of the individual studies, however, did consider lycopene levels in the blood. The analysis noted that the protective effect was slightly stronger for cooked tomato products and that small amounts of added fat improved lycopene absorption. On the other hand, **2 studies from 2007, one of about 1,500 men and the second of more than 28,000 men, found no difference in blood lycopene levels between those in whom**

prostate cancer later developed and those in whom it did not. Such mixed results sometimes happen when there is no effect or only a small effect from the substance being looked at. (American Cancer.org)

There have been several experimental studies on the role of lycopene in preventing or treating cancer. **One animal study found that lycopene treatment reduced the growth of brain tumors. Another animal study showed that frequent intake of lycopene over a long period of time considerably suppressed breast tumor growth in mice.** But breast cancer in humans is very different from breast cancer in mice, and those results may not apply to the disease in humans. **There has been a human study that assigned men at high risk for prostate cancer to take an ordinary multivitamin either with or without a lycopene supplement. This study found no difference in prostate-specific antigen (PSA, a marker of prostate cancer) levels between the 2 groups.** Further studies are needed to find out if any possible anti-cancer properties could benefit humans.

Since tomatoes also contain vitamins, potassium, and other carotenoids and antioxidants, **it may be that other compounds in tomatoes may account for some of the protective effects first thought to be due to lycopene.**

These compounds may act alone or along with lycopene. When researchers look at large population groups with different lifestyles and habits, **it is also possible that their findings can be explained by other factors that were not examined.**

To test whether lycopene is the main cancer-fighting substance in tomatoes, one animal study compared lycopene supplements to powdered tomatoes. Groups of rats who were fed tomato powder were compared to rats given lycopene. **The rats that received tomato powder had much lower cancer risk, whereas the rats receiving lycopene supplements did not differ significantly from the group that received no special supplements.** (Boileau et al, 2003)

A controlled study in a small group of men with prostate cancer found that **lycopene supplements appeared to reduce the rapid growth of prostate cancer cells.** However, **a more recent study with men whose prostate cancer had stopped responding to hormone therapy found that lycopene did not have a significant effect.**

One short-term study from 2006 reported that lycopene sup-plements were safe, but that they did not lower the levels of prostate-specific antigen (a marker of prostate cancer) in men with prostate cancer that had come back. Another reported that the combination of lycopene and soy supplements prevented PSA lev-els from increasing in some men with prostate cancer. (Campbell et al, 2004) (Clark et al, 2006) (Doyle et al, 2006)

The few clinical trials that have been completed have reported mainly the short-term effects on the level of PSA in the blood, which is gener-ally considered a good indicator of prostate cancer growth. Although these studies are an important step, they are not as valuable as long-term studies that look at whether a treatment actually helps patients live longer or relieves their symptoms.

References on lycopene and prostate cancer are as follows: (Norrish et al, 2000) (Paiva, Russell, 1999) (Peters, Leitzmann et al, 2007) (Vaishampayan et al, 2007) (Haseen et al, 2009) (Jatoi et al, 2007) (Kirsh, Mayne et al, 2006) (NCI, 2010)

Most of the human studies that have been published so far were case control studies or other observational studies, which are more prone to error than clinical trials are. More in-formation from clinical trials (including results of several studies already under way) will be needed to be sure whether lycopene-rich foods can help prevent or treat cancer. There are also studies to find out if there are other benefits from lycopene.

Choosing foods from a variety of fruits, vegetables, and other plant sources such as nuts, seeds, whole grains, and beans is likely to be healthier than eating large amounts of one type of food. The American Cancer Society's most recent nutrition guidelines recom-mend eating a balanced diet with an emphasis on plant sources, which includes:

- 5 or more servings of vegetables and fruit each day

- choosing whole grains over processed and refined grains

- limiting processed meats and red meats

- balancing calorie intake with physical activity to get to or stay at a healthy weight

- limiting alcohol intake

- Based on today's evidence, the foods you eat are likely to play a greater role in preventing cancer than in treating it.

Are there any possible problems or complications?

This product is sold as a dietary supplement in the United States. Unlike drugs (which must be tested before being allowed to be sold), the companies that make supplements are not required to prove to the Food and Drug Administration that their supplements are safe or effective, as long as they don't claim the supplements can prevent, treat, or cure any specific disease.

Some such products may not contain the amount of the herb or substance that is written on the label, and some may include other substances (contaminants). Actual amounts per dose may vary between brands or even between different batches of the same brand. The FDA has written new rules to improve the quality of manufacturing processes for dietary supplements and the accurate listing of supplement ingredients. But, the new rules do not address the safety of supplement ingredients or their effects on health when proper manufacturing techniques are used.

Most such supplements have not been tested to find out if they interact with medicines, foods, or other herbs and supplements. Even though some reports of interactions and harmful effects may be published, full studies of interactions and effects are not often available. Because of these limitations, any information on ill effects and interactions below should be considered incomplete.

Lycopene obtained from eating fruits and vegetables has no known side effects and is thought to be safe for humans. The potential side effects of lycopene supplements are not fully known. **Patients in one study who took a lycopene-rich tomato supplement of 15 milligrams twice a day had some intestinal side effects such as nausea, vomiting, diarrhea, indigestion, gas, and bloating.** When consumed over a long period of time, very large amounts of tomato products can give the skin an orange color.

Supplements containing antioxidants such as lycopene may interfere with radiation therapy and chemotherapy if taken during cancer treatment. Even though studies have not been done in humans, antioxidants are known to clean up free radicals, which could interfere with one of the methods by which chemotherapy and radiation destroy cancer cells. Eating fruits and vegetables high in antioxidants is still considered safe during cancer treatment. (Lawenda et al, 2008)

Relying on this type of treatment alone and avoiding or delaying conventional medical care for cancer may have serious health consequences.

Overview

People who have diets rich in tomatoes, which contain lycopene, appear in some studies to have a lower risk of certain types of cancer, especially cancers of the prostate, lung, and stomach. However, **not all of the studies have reached the same conclusion. Studies that tested lycopene on men who already had prostate cancer have been mixed, but in general found little effect.**

Further research is needed to find out what role, if any, lycopene has in the prevention or treatment of cancer.

It is likely that the preventive effect of diets high in fruits and vegetables cannot be explained by just one single part of the diet.

Mayo Clinic Lycopene General Information

http://www.mayoclinic.org/drugs-supplements/lycopene/evidence/hrb-20059666

Mayo Clinic website discussion of lycopene:

Is lycopene a good antioxidant? Although lycopene is believed to have antioxidant benefits, **human research has found mixed results in this area**. Most trials looked at lycopene levels in the body or focused on tomatoes or tomato-based products, rather than on lycopene supplements. Although the limited studies on lycopene supplements suggest antioxidant benefits, many products used contained mixed ingredients.

Can lycopene effectively treat asthma? A number of studies suggest that lycopene may have antioxidant benefits. These effects are believed to help prevent asthma caused by exercise, although the method is still unclear. **Early studies also report that tomato-rich diets may benefit people with asthma.** However, available research has used products and supplements with mixed ingredients.

Is lycopene a blood thinner? Although it has not been well studied in humans, **early research suggests that lycopene may act as a blood thinner**. Most available research in humans has been limited to the use of tomato extract.

Does lycopene aid in chemotherapy of brain tumors? There is limited research on the use of lycopene together with chemotherapy for brain tumors. Early research suggests that this combination may lack significant benefit over chemotherapy alone.

Can lycopene prevent breast cancer? Lycopene and lycopene-rich foods have been studied as a potential therapy for breast cancer. Early studies on breast cancer recurrence and prevention have looked for a possible link between disease risk and fruit or vegetable intake, tomato consumption, or lycopene levels, with mixed results. There is a lack of studies on lycopene supplementation in breast cancer prevention.

Can lycopene be used as an overall cancer preventative? Some studies suggest that fruit and vegetable-rich diets may be linked to reduced cancer risk. Although it has not been well studied in humans, **early research suggests that lycopene may help prevent a number of different cancers, including bladder cancer and skin cancer**. However, the reason behind this potential benefit remains unclear. Studies have also looked at the potential role of tomatoes, tomato-based products, and lycopene levels, but not lycopene supplements. **At this time, strong evidence in support of lycopene for preventing cancer is lacking.**

Can lycopene prevent cervical cancer? Research has looked at the possible use of lycopene in preventing cervical cancer. **Some studies on tomato intake, lycopene levels, and disease risk suggest that lycopene intake may have significant benefit**. However, **others have found conflicting results**.

Can lycopene be used in the treatment of coronary artery disease? A number of studies suggest that higher lycopene levels may be linked to lower risk of coronary artery disease. These benefits are thought to be due to lycopene's antioxidant effects. It has also been suggested that antioxidants like lycopene may reduce the risk of disease progression. However, **results are still mixed, and most studies use mixed ingredient therapies.**

Can lycopene be used in the treatment of type-2 diabetes? **Evidence in support of a link between lycopene or lycopene-containing foods and type 2 diabetes risk is currently lacking.** In human research, evidence is also lacking to support a benefit of tomato supplementation on a therapeutic effect of long-term tomato supplementation on blood sugar levels in people with type 2 diabetes.

Can lycopene be used against prostate cancer? Lycopene has been studied for the prevention of prostate cancer, with **mixed results**. Early research suggests that **lycopene supplementation may slow disease progression associated with enlarged prostate**. Most studies looking at the effects of lycopene on prostate cancer have focused on tomato consumption and have found mixed results. While some research suggests a significant link between lycopene intake from tomatoes with reduced prostate cancer risk, others reported **conflicting findings**.

Can lycopene help treat eye disorders or gum disease? Lycopene has been suggested as a possible treatment for some eye disorders. These include age-related macular degeneration (AMD), which is a breakdown of the retina that may lead to vision loss and cataracts, or clouding of the lens, in the eye. **Results from early studies have been mostly negative.** Although some studies suggest that there may be a link between higher lycopene levels and reduced risk of cataracts or AMD, there are conflicting results. Early evidence reports that a mixed ingredient preparation that contains lycopene and other nutrients found in whole tomatoes may help reduce gum disease, bleeding, and plaque.

Can lycopene be used to prevent lung cancer? Several studies suggest that increased lycopene intake may reduce the risk of lung cancer. **Others report a possible link between consumption of yellow-orange vegetables and lung cancer, as well as lycopene levels and lung cancer**. However, there are conflicting results suggesting that lycopene intake or levels may lack benefit in terms of lung cancer development. Due to the lack of consistency among studies, a conclusion is unable to be made at this time.

Can lycopene lower low-density lipoprotein cholesterol and total cholesterol? Available research suggests that doses of more than 25 milligrams of lycopene daily may lower levels of low-density lipoprotein (LDL, or "bad") cholesterol and total cholesterol.

Can lycopene be used against kidney disease and cancer? High-quality studies on the use of lycopene supplementation for kidney disorders or cancer are lacking. **Early research suggests that lycopene may lack significant benefit in terms of reducing kidney cell cancer.**

Can lycopene be used against inflammation? Early research suggests **that lycopene from a mixed ingredient supplement or from fresh tomatoes may lack anti-inflammatory benefits**. Results have been inconsistent between studies, many of which have looked at mixed-ingredient therapies.

Can lycopene correct oxidative damage to sperm? It has been suggested that oxidative damage may negatively affect sperm. Lycopene is believed to have antioxidant benefits and has been studied for use in infertility. Although a link between lycopene levels and semen quality has been suggested, **studies in humans have found conflicting results**.

Can lycopene treat high blood pressure? Lycopene has been studied for its potential protective effects on the heart. However, the results are mixed. **While some studies report that lycopene may help lower blood pressure, others suggest a lack of benefit or association between lycopene levels and high blood pressure risk**. Most of the therapies studied have contained mixed ingredients. Early research has found inconsistent results on the use of lycopene in preventing high blood pressure in pregnancy, eclampsia. **One trial reported a lack of effect, while another reported reduced risk of high blood pressure in pregnancy and fetal growth problems in women having their first child**. Most studies looked at mixed-ingredient supplements, and the effects of lycopene alone need to be determined.

Can lycopene treat heart disease? **Early research in humans has found mixed results on the possible link between tomato products and a reduced risk of heart disease. Strong evidence in support of this benefit is lacking.**

Can lycopene offer sun protection? The use of lycopene together with other nutrients such as beta-carotene, vitamin C, and vitamin E has been suggested as a possible way to protect skin from sun damage. Lycopene-rich tomato paste has also been suggested as a sun protection method. Although benefits have been seen in small studies, more research is needed before a firm conclusion may be made.

Can lycopene prevent upper gastrointestinal and colorectal cancer? There is inconclusive evidence in support of lycopene for use in preventing cancers of the digestive tract. Limited research reports that there may be a significant decrease in cancer risk with high tomato intake. However, other studies have found either a lack of evidence or conflicting results for stomach and colorectal cancer.

Is lycopene an immune stimulant? The effect of beta-carotene on immune function has been studied, but research on other similar pigments is limited. **A small number of trials on lycopene consumption found a lack of benefit for this purpose.**

Although information is limited, there is enough evidence available to conclude a lack of effectiveness.

Prof Randolph M Howes MD,PhD

Nov 1, 2013 ... Although lycopene is believed to have antioxidant benefits, human research has found mixed results in this area.

LYCOPENE

Lycopene is a **powerful antioxidant** found in tomatoes and pink grapefruit.

Like the better-known supplement beta-carotene, lycopene belongs to the family of chemicals known as *carotenoids*. As an antioxidant, it is about twice as powerful as beta-carotene.

Sources

Lycopene is not a necessary or essential nutrient.

However, like other substances found in fruits and vegetables, some believe that it may be very important for optimal health.

Tomatoes are the best source of lycopene.

Fortunately, **cooking doesn't destroy lycopene**, so pizza sauce is just as good as a fresh tomato.

In fact, **some studies indicate that cooking tomatoes in oil may provide lycopene in a way that the body can use better**, (Weisburger, 1998) (Sies, Stahl, 1998) **although not all studies agree**. (Rao, Agarwal, 1998)

Lycopene is also found in watermelon, guava, and pink grapefruit. Synthetic, supplemental lycopene is also available and appears to be as well absorbed as natural-source lycopene.

Therapeutic Dosages

The optimum dosage for lycopene has not been established, but the amount found helpful in studies generally fell in the range of 4 to 8 mg daily.

It has been suggested the lycopene is better absorbed when it is taken with fats such as olive oil, but one study failed to find any meaningful change in absorption.

Therapeutic Uses

Claims: Some but not all observational studies suggest that foods containing lycopene may help prevent macular degeneration, cataracts, cardiovascular disease and cancer.

However, **observational studies are highly unreliable means of determining the effectiveness of medical treatments**; only double-blind studies can do so, and few have been performed that relate to the potential uses of lycopene.

Investigators evaluated the effect of pre-natal supplementation of anti-oxidant Lycopene in prevention of pre-eclampsia in the high risk pregnant women. Of the total of 54 women, 30 women were **randomized** to receive Lycopene in a dose of 2 mg twice daily starting from the date of entry and were instructed to continue the drug regularly until delivery. The other 24 women were randomized to the control group and they did not take lycopene. **Lycopene supplementation does not decrease the incidence of preeclampsia in high risk women**. (Antartani, Ashok, 2011)

However despite these promising results researchers are cautious about drawing conclusions: several other nutritional substances have shown promise for preventing preeclampsia in preliminary trials **only to fail when larger and more definitive studies were done**. (Sibai, 1998)

Lycopene has also shown promise for leukoplakia, a precancerous condition of the mouth and other mucous membranes. In a **double-blind, placebo-controlled study, 58 people with oral leukoplakia** received either 8 mg oral lycopene daily, 4 mg daily, or placebo capsules for three months. Participants were then followed for an additional two months. The results indicated that **lycopene in either dose was more effective than placebo for reducing signs and symptoms of leukoplakia, and that 8 mg daily was more effective than 4 mg.**

Lycopene (taken at a dose of 16 g daily) has shown promise for oral submucous fibrosis, a severe condition of the mouth primarily associated with excessive chewing of betel nuts.

Regarding yet another mouth condition, gingivitis (periodontal disease), **the results of a small double-blind trial suggest that lycopene can offers benefits when taken on its own, or when used to augment the effectiveness of standard care.** (Chandra et al, 2007)

Much weaker evidence—far too weak to rely upon at all—hints that lycopene or a standardized tomato extract containing lycopene might be helpful for treating a number of conditions, including prostate cancer, hypertension, breast cancer and male infertility, and for preventing heart disease, sunburn, and testicular damage caused by the cancer chemotherapy drug adriamycin.

Weak evidence hints that lycopene might help protect against side-effects caused by the drug doxorubicin, specifically damage to the heart and to developing sperm cells.

Results of studies have been **inconsistent** regarding the effects of lycopene and exercise-induced asthma. (Falk et al, 2995) (Neuman et al, 2000)

One observational study failed to find that high consumption of lycopene reduced risk of developing diabetes. (Wang et al, 2006)

Safety Issues

Lycopene is believed to be a safe supplement, as evidenced by the fact that researchers felt comfortable giving it to pregnant women. One evaluation of the literature concluded that long term use of lycopene should be generally safe in doses up to at least 75 mg per day.

Note: We suggest that pregnant women should consult with a physician before taking any herbs or supplements.

Maximum safe dosages for young children, pregnant or nursing women, or those with severe liver or kidney disease have not been established.

No Magic Tomato?

Study breaks link between lycopene and prostate cancer prevention.

5-17-07

Tomatoes might be nutritious and tasty, but don't count on them to prevent prostate cancer. In the **May 2007 issue of Cancer Epidemiology, Biomarkers & Prevention**, researchers based at the National Cancer Institute and Fred Hutchinson Cancer Research Center report that

lycopene, an antioxidant predominately found in tomatoes, does not effectively prevent prostate cancer.

In fact, the researchers noted an association between beta-carotene, an antioxidant related to lycopene, and an increased risk for aggressive prostate cancer.

According to the researchers, the study is one of the largest to evaluate the role of blood concentrations of lycopene and other carotenoid antioxidants in preventing prostate cancer. Study data were derived from over **28,000 men enrolled in the Prostate, Lung, Colorectal, and Ovarian (PLCO) Cancer Screening Trial**, an ongoing, **randomized National Cancer Institute trial** to evaluate cancer screening methods and to investigate early markers of cancer.

"It is disappointing, since lycopene might have offered a simple and inexpensive way to lower prostate cancer risk for men concerned about this common disease," said **Ulrike Peters, Ph.D., M.P.H., of the Fred Hutchinson Cancer Research Center.** "Unfortunately, this easy answer just does not work."

Previous studies suggested that a diet rich in lycopene protected against prostate cancer, spurring commercial and public interest in the antioxidant. Antioxidants protect against free radicals, highly reactive atoms and molecules that can damage DNA and other important molecules in the cell. Since free radical damage increases with age, there has been **a long-held suspicion** in the scientific community that free radical damage could increase the risk of prostate cancer, a disease that has been clearly associated with age.

Subsequent studies of the potentially protective role of lycopene have been contradictory or inconclusive, according to Peters. **In a 2006 study, she and her colleagues looked at the dietary intake of more than 25 tomato-based foods, also using data from the PLCO trial, and found no overall association between lycopene intake and prostate cancer.**

In their current study, the researchers followed over 28,000 men between the ages of 55 and 74, enrolled in the PLCO Trial, with no history of prostate cancer. The men were initially screened through a PSA test and digital rectal exam, and were then followed through routine exams and screenings until first occurrence of prostate cancer, death or the end of the trial in 2001. At the beginning of the trial, the men gave a blood sample and completed a questionnaire related to their health, diet and lifestyle.

The researchers focused on non-Hispanic Caucasian men, as the small number of cases among other ethnic groups was statistically insignificant. **They found no significant difference between those who had prostate cancer and those who did not in relation to the concentration of lycopene in their bloodstream. "Our results do not offer support for the benefits of lycopene against prostate cancer,"** Peters said.

Most surprisingly, says Peters, was the relationship between increased risk of aggressive prostate cancer – defined as disease that has spread beyond the prostate – and beta-carotene, another antioxidant found in many vegetables and commonly used as a dietary supplement. This increased risk of aggressive prostate cancer is also found with omega-3 fish oil

This unexpected observation "may be due to chance, however **beta carotene is already known to increase risk of lung cancer and cardiovascular disease in smokers**," Peters said.

"While it would be counter-productive to advise people against eating carrots and leafy vegetables, I would say to **be cautious about taking beta carotene supplements, particularly at high doses,** and consult a physician," Peters said.

Lycopene ($C_{40}H_{56}$) is a natural fat-soluble pigment found in plants where it serves as an accessory light-gathering pigment and free radical quencher. This carotenoid is an open chain polyisoprenoid with 11 conjugated double bonds. Lycopene occurs in food sources predominantly as all-*trans*-lycopene. Various *cis*-isomers also are found in human blood and tissues, suggesting post-ingestive isomerization.

Because lycopene is acyclic it does not serve as a substrate for ß-carotene 15,15'-dioxygenase and therefore cannot be converted to vitamin A.

Double-blind, placebo-controlled studies are the gold standard for determining effectiveness of a treatment. Only a few ingredients have some direct clinical evidence (from double-blind clinical trials) to support their use in for cancer prevention: green tea, lycopene, selenium and, possibly, vitamin E. However, even in these cases the evidence remains far from conclusive.

Lycopene: **Preliminary research has raised concerns that lycopene might worsen established prostate cancer by increasing metastasis.**

Latest Prostate Cancer News
http://www.prostate-cancer.org/pcricms/node/311?id=40161

Little Evidence Lycopene Reduces Cancer Risk

According to a review conducted by the U.S. Food and Drug Administration (FDA), there is "no credible evidence" that lycopene reduces the risk of cancers such as prostate cancer, and "very limited evidence" that tomato consumption reduces risk. The review was published in the *Journal of the National Cancer Institute.*

Lycopene is a carotenoid found in tomatoes and other red fruits. Some studies have suggested that lycopene or lycopene-containing foods such as tomatoes may reduce the risk of certain types of cancer, particularly prostate cancer. **Other studies, however, have failed to find a link.**

In response to groups who wanted to make claims about the cancer benefits of lycopene or tomatoes, in 2007, **the FDA conducted a review of the available scientific evidence.** The main conclusions of the review were the following:

- **There is no credible evidence that lycopene reduces the risk of prostate, lung, colorectal, gastric, breast, ovarian, endometrial, or pancreatic cancer.**

- **There is no credible evidence that tomato consumption reduces the risk of lung, colorectal, breast, cervical, or endometrial cancer.**

- **There is very limited evidence that tomato consumption reduces the risk of prostate, ovarian, gastric, and pancreatic cancer.**

(Kavanaugh et al, 2007)

In an accompanying editorial, Dr. Edward Giovannucci addressed possible reasons for the inconsistent results of previous studies. (Giovannucci, 2007)

Dr. Giovannucci participated in several of the studies that reported a protective effect of lycopene and/or tomato products against prostate cancer.

Noting that lycopene or tomatoes may reduce the risk of cancer progression (rather than cancer initiation), Dr. Giovannucci explained that studies conducted recently—after the widespread adoption of PSA testing—may miss an effect of lycopene. Prostate cancers detected by PSA testing tend to be very early-stage; furthermore, some of the cancers detected by PSA testing are likely to be indolent, slow-growing cancers. If lycopene acts later in the process of prostate cancer development, when a cancer is progressing to a more aggressive or advanced stage, a study that includes mainly PSA-detected cancers may fail to detect this effect. This remains speculative however.

Dr. Giovannucci concluded: "Although it may be premature to espouse increased consumption of tomato sauce or lycopene for prostate cancer prevention, this area of research remains promising."

Ineffectiveness of lycopene and curcumin on rat prostate carcer

The chemopreventive efficacy of lycopene and curcumin with regard to prostate carcinogenesis was investigated using 3,2'-dimethyl-4-aminobiphenol (DMAB)- and 2-amino-1-methylimidazo[4,5-b]pyridine (PhIP)-induced rat ventral prostate cancer models. Three 60 week experiments with male F344 rats were carried out. In the first DMAB was given for the first 20 weeks and lycopene or curcumin were administered concomitantly or subsequently at dietary doses of 15 and 500 p.p.m., respectively. In the second experiment lycopene and curcumin were given to rats pretreated with DMAB at doses of 5, 15 or 45 p.p.m. or 100 or 500 p.p.m. In the third PhIP was selected as an initiator for prostate carcinogenesis and administered for 20 weeks. Rats were then fed a diet containing lycopene at a dose of 45 p.p.m. or curcumin at a dose of 500 p.p.m. or both together. Chemopreventive effects of lycopene and curcumin on development of DMAB-induced ventral prostate carcinomas were observed only in the first experiment and no confirmation of inhibition potential was obtained in the following studies. Neither summational nor synergistic chemoprevention was evident. It is concluded from the present data that, **overall, neither lycopene nor curcumin can consistently prevent rat prostate carcinogenesis.** (Imaida et al, 2001)

Lycopene at a dose as low as 0.5 p.p.m. has been reported to inhibit appearance of spontaneous mammary tumors. (Nagasawa et al, 1995)

However, **there are also some studies that failed to demonstrate anticancer efficacy of lycopene in the liver, colon, urinary bladder and lung.** (Kim et al, 1997) (Okajima et al, 1997) (Hect et al, 1999) (Cohen et al, 1999)

Dietary and blood carotenoids, including alpha-carotene, beta-carotene, lycopene, lutein/zeaxanthin, and beta-cryptoxanthin, have been examined in a number of epidemiological studies in recent years for the risk of cardiovascular disease. This review assimilated the existing and recent literature on carotenoids and cardiovascular disease and considered what research gaps may remain.

RECENT FINDINGS: Numerous large cohort studies have been published in largely American men and women that have examined dietary intake or blood levels of total or individual carotenoids with the risk of various cardiovascular endpoints. *Overall, early, promising results have grown increasingly inconsistent over time.*

More recently, studies examining lycopene and lutein/zeaxanthin have offered more promising data on a possible, but not yet established, inverse association with the risk of cardiovascular disease. Recent epidemiological data on beta-cryptoxanthin and cardiovascular disease are lacking.

Primary and secondary prevention trials have extensively examined beta-carotene, but not other carotenoids, for the risk of cardiovascular disease as either the primary or secondary endpoint with largely null results. More recent studies have focused on individual carotenoids in relation to cardiovascular disease and require a more careful evaluation of potential mechanisms of effect.

SUMMARY

The promise of early epidemiological studies on carotenoids and cardiovascular disease paved the way to largely disappointing results from several large prevention trials of beta-carotene.

Emerging recent evidence of potential cardioprotective effects for lycopene and other carotenoids besides beta-carotene in the diet and blood suggest that there is more to be learned in the story of carotenoids and both atherosclerotic progression and clinically manifested cardiovascular disease. (Sesso, 2006)

Prof Randolph M Howes MD,PhD

Dark chocolate or tomato extract for prehypertension: an RCT

Abstract

BACKGROUND:

Flavanol-rich chocolate and lycopene-rich tomato extract have attracted interest as potential alternative treatment options for hypertension, a known risk factor for cardiovascular morbidity and mortality. Treatment of prehypertension (SBP 120-139/DBP 80-89 mmHg) may forestall progression to hypertension. However, there has been only limited research into non-pharmacological treatment options for prehypertension. We investigated the effect of dark chocolate or tomato extract on blood pressure, and their acceptability as an ongoing treatment option in a prehypertensive population.

METHODS:

Our trial consisted of two phases: a randomized controlled three group-parallel trial over 12 weeks (phase 1) followed by a crossover of the two active treatment arms over an additional 12-week period (phase 2). **Group 1 received a 50 g daily dose of dark chocolate with 70% cocoa containing 750 mg polyphenols**, group 2 were allocated one tomato extract capsule containing 15 mg lycopene per day, and group 3 received one placebo capsule daily over 8 weeks followed by a 4-week washout period. In phase 2 the active treatment groups were crossed over to receive the alternative treatment. Median blood pressure, weight, and abdominal circumference were measured 4-weekly, and other characteristics including physical activity, general health, energy, mood, and acceptability of treatment were assessed by using a linear mixed model, and one time point differences using Kruskal-Wallis, Fisher's-Exact, or t-tests.

RESULTS:

Thirty-six prehypertensive healthy adult volunteers completed the 6-month trial. Blood pressure changes over time within groups and between groups were not signifi cant and independent of treatment. **Weight and other characteristics did not change significantly during the trial**. However, a marked difference in acceptability between the two treatment forms (chocolate or capsule) was revealed (p < 0.0001). Half of the participants allocated to the chocolate treatment found it hard to eat 50 g of dark chocolate every day and 20% considered it an unacceptable long-term treatment option, whereas all participants found it easy and acceptable to take a capsule each day for blood pressure.

CONCLUSION:

Our study did not find a blood pressure lowering effect of dark chocolate or tomato extract in a prehypertensive population. Practicability of chocolate as a long-term treatment option may be limited. (Reid et al, 2009)

General information on lycopene

Lycopene is a naturally occurring chemical that gives fruits and vegetables a red color. It is one of a number of pigments called carotenoids. Lycopene is found in watermelons, pink grapefruits, apricots, and pink guavas. It is found in particularly high amounts in tomatoes and tomato products.

In North America, 85% of dietary lycopene comes from tomato products such as tomato juice or paste. One cup (240 mL) of tomato juice provides about 23 mg of lycopene.

Processing raw tomatoes using heat (in the making of tomato juice, tomato paste or ketchup, for example) actually changes the lycopene in the raw product into a form that is easier for the body to use. The lycopene in supplements is about as easy for the body to use as lycopene found in food.

People take lycopene for preventing heart disease, "hardening of the arteries" (atherosclerosis); and cancer of the prostate, breast, lung, bladder, ovaries, colon, and pancreas.

Lycopene is also used for treating human papilloma virus (HPV) infection, which is a major cause of uterine cancer. Some people also use lycopene for cataracts and asthma.

How does it work?

Lycopene is a powerful antioxidant that may help protect cells from damage. This is why there is a lot of research interest in lycopene's role, if any, in preventing cancer.

Lycopene is considered ineffective in preventing diabetes. And, according to WebMD, there is insufficient evidence for the following:

- **Prostate cancer.** Early research in men with precancerous changes in their prostate shows that taking 4 mg of lycopene supplements twice daily might delay or prevent progression to prostate cancer. In addition, researchers have surveyed men about their diet and health and found contradictory information about a possible role for lycopene in preventing prostate cancer. Some of these studies show that lycopene from foods, such as tomato products, is associated with a lower risk of developing prostate cancer. **But other research shows no association between dietary lycopene intake and prostate cancer risk.** However, for men in this study who had a family history of prostate cancer, getting more lycopene from food seemed to offer some protection against getting prostate cancer.

- **Breast cancer.** Several studies have tried to determine whether getting more lycopene from food or taking supplements will help to prevent breast cancer. But **findings have not agreed**.

- **Bladder cancer.** Research to date suggests that lycopene intake from the diet and lycopene levels in the blood **don't affect the risk of getting bladder cancer**.

- **Ovarian cancer.** Some research shows that a diet rich in **carotenoids, including lycopene, seems to help prevent ovarian cancer in young (premenopausal) women**.

- **Pancreatic cancer.** Some research shows that **a diet high in lycopene, primarily from tomatoes, seems to lower the risk of getting pancreatic cancer**. This is far from proven.

- **Lung cancer.** There is **some evidence** that getting lycopene from foods -- 12 mg/day or more for men, and 6.5 mg/day or more for women—**lowers lung cancer risk** in nonsmoking men aged 40 to 75, and nonsmoking women aged 30 to 55.

- **Cancer of the colon and rectum.** Research so far suggests that there is **no connection between dietary lycopene and the risk of getting cancer of the colon or rectum.**

- **White pre-cancerous patches in the mouth (oral leukoplakia).** Developing clinical research shows that taking 8 mg/day or 4 mg/day of a specific lycopene supplement (LycoRed, Jagsonpal Pharmaceutical) **significantly improves oral leukoplakia.**

- **Heart disease.** Study results are mixed. **Some research shows that women with higher levels of lycopene in their blood have a lower risk of getting heart disease. But other studies show no link between lycopene intake and the risk of heart attack and stroke in women. In men already at low risk for heart disease, increasing dietary lycopene does not seem to prevent heart attacks.**

- **Eye disease** (age related maculopathy). So far, it appears that **dietary lycopene has no effect on getting or preventing age-related maculopathy (AMD).**

- **Human papilloma virus (HPV)** infection. **Women with higher levels of lycopene in their blood seem to get over HPV infections.**

- "Hardening of the arteries" (atherosclerosis).

- Asthma attacks brought on by exercise.

- Cataracts.

- Other conditions.

More evidence is needed to rate lycopene for these uses.

Warnings of possible adverse effects are as follows:

Lycopene is **LIKELY SAFE** when taken by mouth in appropriate amounts. Daily supplements containing 30 mg of lycopene have been used safely for up to 8 weeks.

Special Precautions & Warnings

Pregnancy and breast-feeding: Lycopene is **LIKELY SAFE** when taken in amounts commonly found in foods. However, not enough is known about the safety of using lycopene supplements during pregnancy or breast-feeding. **If you are pregnant or breast-feeding, avoid using lycopene in amounts greater than those typically found in foods.**

Prostate cancer: Developing laboratory research suggests ly-copene might worsen established prostate cancer by increas-ing the spread of cancer without having any effect on cancer cell growth. Until more is known, avoid lycopene if you have a pros-tate cancer diagnosis.

The appropriate dose of lycopene depends on several factors such as the user's age, health, and several other conditions. **At this time in 2009, there is not enough scientific information to determine an appropriate range of doses for lycopene**.

Keep in mind that natural products are not always necessarily safe and dosages can be important. Be sure to follow relevant directions on product labels and consult your pharmacist or physician or other healthcare professional before using.

'Tomato pill' hope for stopping heart disease

6-9-10

Taking a tomato pill a day could help keep heart disease at bay, say UK scientists who have carried out a small but robust study.

The trial, which tested the tomato pill versus a dummy drug in **72 adults, found it improved the functioning of blood vessels.**

But experts say more studies are needed to prove it really works.

The pill contains **lycopene, a natural antioxidant that also gives tomatoes their color**.

Experts have suspected for some time that lycopene might be good for avoiding illnesses, including certain cancers and cardiovascular disease.

There is some evidence that eating a Mediterranean-style diet, which is rich in tomatoes (as well as other fruit and vegetables and olive oil), is beneficial for health.

Following a healthy diet is still advisable but scientists have been re-searching whether there is a way to put at least some of this good stuff into an easy-to-take pill.

Tomato pill of CamNutra

A company called **CamNutra has come up with its own "tomato pill"**.

Working independently of CamNutra, and instead **funded by the Wellcome Trust, the British Heart Foundation and the National Institute of Health Research, a team at Cambridge University set out to see if this pill would have the desired effect**.

They recruited 36 volunteers known to have heart disease and 36 "healthy" controls, who were all given a daily tablet to take, which was either the tomato pill or a placebo. To ensure a fairer trial, neither the volunteers nor the researchers were told what the tablets actually contained until after the two-month study had ended and the results were in.

For comparison, the researchers measured something called **forearm blood flow**, which is predictive of future cardiovascular risk because narrowed blood vessels can lead to heart attack and stroke.

In the heart disease patients, the tomato pill improved forearm blood flow significantly, while the placebo did not.

The supplement had no effect on blood pressure, arterial stiffness or levels of fats in the blood, however.

- A natural antioxidant - substances thought to protect the body's cells from damage

- Found in tomatoes, but also in apricots, watermelon and papaya as well as pink grapefruit

- Lycopene content varies according to the variety of tomato and how it is prepared e.g., puree, ketchup, cooked or raw

- It is unclear whether supplements would ever be able to replace the benefits of a varied diet

Lead researcher Dr Joseph Cheriyan said the findings, published in PLoS One journal, were promising, but added: "A daily 'tomato pill' is not a substitute for other treatments, but may provide added benefits when taken alongside other medication.

"However, we cannot answer if this may reduce heart disease - this would need much larger trials to investigate outcomes more carefully."

Prof Jeremy Pearson of the British Heart Foundation said big studies were needed to see if this could become a viable option for patients.

Genetically-modified purple tomatoes heading for shops

1-6-14

The new tomatoes could improve the nutritional value of everyday foods. The prospect of genetically modified purple tomatoes reaching the shelves has come a step closer.

Their dark pigment is intended to give tomatoes the same potential health benefits as fruit such as blueberries.

Developed in Britain, large-scale production is now under way in Canada with the first 1,200 liters of purple tomato juice ready for shipping.

The pigment, known as **anthocyanin, is an antioxidant which studies on animals show could help fight cancer.**

Scientists say the new tomatoes could improve the nutritional value of everything from **ketchup to pizza topping.**

The tomatoes were developed at the John Innes Centre in Norwich where Prof Cathie Martin hopes the first delivery of large quantities of juice will allow researchers to investigate its potential.

"With these purple tomatoes you can get the same compounds that are present in blueberries and cranberries that give them their health benefits - but you can apply them to foods that people actually eat in significant amounts and are reasonably affordable," she said.

"I hope this will serve as a vanguard product where people can have access to something that is GM but has benefits for them," end Quote Prof Cathie Martin John Innes Centre in Norwich.

The tomatoes are part of a new generation of GM plants designed to appeal to consumers - the first types were aimed specifically at farmers as new tools in agriculture.

The purple pigment is the result of the transfer of a gene from a snapdragon plant - the modification triggers a process within the tomato plant allowing the anthocyanin to develop.

Although the invention is British, Prof Martin says European Union restrictions on GM encouraged her to look abroad to develop the technology.

Canadian regulations are seen as more supportive of GM and that led to a deal with an Ontario company, New Energy Farms, which is now producing enough purple tomatoes in a 465 square meter (5,000sq ft) greenhouse to make 2,000 liters (440 gallons) of juice.

According to Prof Martin, the Canadian system is "very enlightened".

"They look at the trait not the technology and that should be a way we **start changing our thinking** - asking if what you're doing is safe and beneficial, not 'Is it GM and therefore we're going to reject it completely'.

"It is frustrating that we've had to go to Canada to do a lot of the growing and the processing and I hope this will serve as a vanguard product where people can have access to something that is GM but has benefits for them."

The first 1,200 liters are due to be shipped to Norwich shortly - and because all the seeds will have been removed, there is no genetic material to risk any contamination.

Scientists at Rothamsted hope to produce a GM plant that provides "fish oil."

The aim is to use the juice in research to conduct a wide range of tests including examining whether the anthocyanin has positive effects on humans. Earlier studies show benefits as an anti-inflammatory and in slowing cancers in mice.

A key question is whether a GM product that may have health benefits will influence public opinion.

A major survey across the European Union in 2010 found opponents outnumbered supporters by roughly three to one. The last approval for a GM food crop in the EU came in 1998.

Prof Martin hopes that **the purple tomato juice will have a good chance of being approved for sale to consumers in North America in as little as two years' time**.

She and other plant researchers in the UK hope that GM will come to be seen in a more positive light.

Legacy of distrust

Earlier on Friday, scientists at Rothamsted Research in Hertfordshire announced that they were seeking permission for field trials for a GM plant that could produce a "fish oil".

In a parallel project, they have been cultivating a type of GM wheat that is designed to release a pheromone that deters aphids.

Professor Nick Pidgeon, an environmental psychologist at Cardiff University, has run opinion polls and focus groups on GM and other technologies.

He says that a legacy of distrust, including from the time of mad cow disease, will cause lasting concern.

"Highlighting benefits will make a difference but it's only one part of the story which is quite complex.

"People will still be concerned that this is a technology that potentially interferes with natural systems - they'll be concerned about big corporations having control over the technology and, at the end of the day, you feed it to yourself and your children and that will be a particular concern for families across the UK."

"To change that quite negative view that people had 10-15 years ago will take quite a long time - it'll take a demonstration of safety, a demonstration of good regulation and of the ability to manage the technology in a safe way. And that doesn't happen overnight."

COMMENT: Foods that are unnatural to human diet, are made more so by genetic vandalism.

My Letter to the Editor: 7-13-11

"Is Lycopene A Cancer Killer?"

Lycopene is the "tomato" antioxidant that is hailed in lay magazines as a possible cure for the prevention of heart disease, cancer of the prostate, breast, lung, bladder, ovaries, colon and pancreas.

Lycopene is also touted as being useful in treating HPV virus infections, which is a major cause of uterine and cervical cancer. Some even claim to use lycopene for treating or preventing cataracts and asthma.

However, all of this must be looked at with an circumspect eye. We must be prudent when considering such outlandish claims and in the end, we must rely on the scientific evidence, not testimonials, opinions or sales pitches.

Lycopene is a natural chemical that gives fruits and vegetables a red color and it has an especially high content in tomatoes. One cup (240 mL) of tomato juice contains about 23 mg of lycopene and the cooking process to make tomato paste or ketchup, changes the lycopene into a form that is more readily useable by the body; whereas, usually, cooking removes some of the helpful components of fresh fruits and vegetables.

Now, let's look at the scientific data.

First, **studies of tomatoes and studies of lycopene are two different things and there is little correlation between the two**.

In 2007, the *Journal of the National Cancer Institute* reported that the FDA conducted a review of the scientific evidence of claims about the cancer benefits of lycopene or tomatoes and concluded:

1) **there is no credible evidence that lycopene reduces the risk of prostate, lung, colorectal, gastric, breast, ovarian, endometrial, or pancreatic cancer**,

2) **there is no credible evidence that tomato consumption reduces the risk of lung, colorectal, breast, cervical, or endometrial cancer**, and

3) **there is very limited evidence that tomato consumption reduces the risk of prostate, ovarian, gastric, and pancreatic cancer**.

Some investigators even suggest that "metabolic products of lycopene, the lycopenoids, may be responsible for some of lycopene's reported bioactivity (not its antioxidant character)."

According to WebMD, developing research suggests that **lycopene may worsen established prostate cancer and they recommend avoiding it if one has a diagnosis of prostate cancer.** However, other sources disagree.

Prof Randolph M Howes MD,PhD

Actually, all men could be considered as being "pre-cancerous" for prostate cancer, because if a man lives long enough, he will likely develop prostate cancer.

We will remain guarded as regards wild, unsupported claims of miraculous cancer cures. We must also remember that supplements do not undergo governmental quality controls and that contaminants are frequently found in them when tested by ConsumerLab.com.

Currently, there is insufficient evidence to draw firm conclusions. Study agents called "validated biomarkers" are tricky and frequently unreliable.

So, lycopene lacks support. Still, I love Creole tomatoes.

Lycopene effects on cardiovascular disease: an RCT

Abstract

AIMS:

The mechanisms by which a 'Mediterranean diet' reduces cardiovascular disease (CVD) burden remain poorly understood. Lycopene is a potent antioxidant found in such diets with evidence suggesting beneficial effects. Investigators studied the effects of lycopene on the vasculature in CVD patients and separately, in healthy volunteers (HV).

METHODS AND RESULTS:

We randomized 36 statin treated CVD patients and 36 healthy volunteers in a $2\alpha1$ treatment allocation ratio to either 7 mg lycopene or placebo daily for 2 months in a double-blind trial. Forearm responses to intra-arterial infusions of acetylcholine (endothelium-dependent vasodilatation; EDV), sodium nitroprusside (endothelium-independent vasodilatation; EIDV), and NG-monomethyl-L-arginine (basal nitric oxide (NO) synthase activity) were measured using venous plethysmography. A range of vascular and biochemical secondary endpoints were also explored. EDV in CVD patients post-lycopene improved by 53% (95% CI: +9% to +93%, P=0.03 vs. placebo) without changes to EIDV, or basal NO responses. **HVs did not show changes in EDV after lycopene treatment. Blood pressure,** arterial stiffness, lipids and hsCRP levels were unchanged for lycopene vs. placebo treatment groups in the CVD arm as well as the HV arm. At baseline, CVD patients had impaired EDV compared with HV (30% lower; 95% CI: -45% to -10%, P=0.008), despite lower LDL cholesterol (1.2 mmol/L lower, 95% CI: -1.6 to -0.9 mmol/L, P<0.001). Post-therapy EDV responses for lycopene-treated CVD patients were similar to HVs at baseline (2% lower, 95% CI: -30% to +30%, P=0.85), also suggesting lycopene improved endothelial function.

CONCLUSIONS

Lycopene supplementation improves endothelial function in CVD patients on optimal secondary prevention, but not in healthy volunteers (HVs). (Gajendragadkar et al, 2014)

Lycopene and heart health

Abstract

Cardiovascular diseases (CVDs) are the leading causes of human morbidity and mortality in developed countries. Specific biomarkers in this context are markers of inflammation, lipid status, thrombosis and oxidative stress. One recommendation for CVD prevention is to increase consumption of fruits and vegetables as good sources of secondary plant products, e.g. carotenoids. This review aimed to show linkages between **lycopene, one main carotenoid in the human diet**, and prevention of heart diseases by looking for epidemiological data, results from in vitro experiments and results from in vivo studies (animal studies and human intervention trials). In addition, patents and products within the context of lycopene and CVD prevention will be discussed with a special emphasis on health claims. Epidemiological data, in vitro data and results from animal experiments partly showed promising preventive mechanisms of lycopene. **In contrast, until now, human intervention studies mostly failed to show any CVD prevention.** However, there is still an encouraging situation, giving hints for antioxidant as well as anti-inflammatory effects of lycopene. These mechanisms could be the background for cardio-protective effects of tomatoes and tomato products. In summary, **there are a lot of investigations needed in the future to give reliable results to establish these CVD-preventive effects.** (Bohm, 2012)

Prof Randolph M Howes MD,PhD

Are the health attributes of lycopene related to its antioxidant function?

Abstract

A variety of epidemiological trials have suggested that higher intake of lycopene-containing foods (primarily tomato products) or blood lycopene concentrations are associated with decreased cardiovascular disease and prostate cancer risk. Of the carotenoids tested, lycopene has been demonstrated to be the most potent in vitro antioxidant leading many researchers to conclude that the antioxidant properties of lycopene are responsible for disease prevention. In our review of human and animal trials with lycopene, or lycopene-containing extracts, **there is limited support for the *in vivo* antioxidant function for lycopene. Moreover, tissue levels of lycopene appear to be too low to play a meaningful antioxidant role.** We conclude that **there is an overall shortage of supportive evidence for the "antioxidant hypothesis" as lycopene's major in vivo mechanism of action.** Our laboratory has postulated that metabolic products of lycopene, **the lycopenoids, may be responsible for some of lycopene's reported bioactivity.** (Erdman, Ford, Lindshield, 2008)

Dietary intake of lycopene, or blood or tissue lycopene, may simply serve as a marker of tomato intake. Lycopene may provide some of the cardiovascular or cancer protection associated with tomato intake, but **likely is not the only bioactive compound in tomatoes.** Tomatoes contain significant quantities of vitamins C and E, folate, polyphenols, and other carotenoids such as phytoene and phytofluene. (Canene-Adams et al, 2005)

Significant concentrations of lycopene are only found in a select number of foods (tomato, watermelon, guava, pink grapefruit), **with about 85% of lycopene intake in the U.S. coming from fresh and processed tomato products.** (Campbell et al, 2004)

In 2000, the panel on Dietary Reference Intakes for Vitamin C, Vitamin E, Selenium and Carotenoids evaluated the potential health impact of β-carotene and other carotenoids. (Anonymous, 2000)

After extensively evaluating the literature, they concluded that there was evidence that β-carotene was an antioxidant *in vitro*, but that there was not convincing evidence that substantially increasing β-carotene intake above current levels had a significant effect on antioxidant status measures. Lycopene was not specifically addressed. However, **the authors of this review have found no compelling evidence since the publication of that panel's report to suggest that elevation of β-carotene or lycopene significantly improves antioxidant status measures.**

There is almost universal agreement that **lycopene is an excellent** *in vitro* **antioxidant, especially in quenching singlet oxygen, and may be the best dietary molecule in this regard**. (Di Mascio et al, 1989)

It is projected that intact **lycopene with its 11 conjugated double bonds** will also quench peroxyl radicals in LDL particles or cellular membranes. (Young et al, 2004)

Carotenoids, while highly concentrated in many foods, are not well absorbed and rarely accumulate in high concentrations in blood and tissues. (Lindshield, Erdman, 2006)

Lycopene is generally the carotenoid in highest concentration in American's serum, nevertheless, the average adult U.S. serum concentrations are less than 0.013 μm/dL according to NHANES III data. It is difficult to exceed 0.14μm/dL lycopene in serum, even when providing a lycopene-enriched diet for a week or more to healthy subjects. These levels fall far short of serum a-tocopherol concentrations.

Some have measured **carotenoid concentrations in human tissues, and lycopene is generally the highest carotenoid in individual tissues**. (Schmitz et al, 1991) (Kaplan et al, 1990)

The following has been excerpted from the Schmitz et al paper:

Sies reminds us that we have an antioxidant enzyme network that constitutes our major defense against oxidative stress. These enzymes intercept ROS and RNS, repair damage to macromolecules, such as DNA, and adapt to changing levels of short and long-term oxidative stress. (Sies et al, 2007) (Sies, Stahl, Sevanian, 2005)

Small molecules such as carotenoids, vitamins, and some minerals contribute to antioxidant defense as part of enzymes (e.g. selenium in glutathione peroxidases, manganese in superoxide dismutase), or play a more direct role by intercepting and/or quenching ROS or RNS (e.g. vitamins E and C). Carotenoids can function as chain-breaking antioxidants.

The quenching of singlet oxygen or peroxyl radicals by carotenoids directly transfers energy between these molecules. (Young et al, 2004)

That energy can be dissipated to the aqueous environment as heat or destroy the carotenoid molecule itself. To be effective antioxidants, carotenoids must be present in sufficient concentrations and at the specific location where the ROS (EMODs) or RNS are generated.

Researchers have postulated that many chronic diseases; cardiovascular disease, cancer, diabetes, eye diseases and aging itself are allegedly the result of long-term oxidative stress.

There is almost universal agreement that consumption of carotenoid-containing fruits and vegetables is associated with decreased incidence of chronic diseases such as heart disease and cancer. It was assumed that carotenoids in these foods are responsible, or at least contribute to these epidemiological findings, but this assumption requires validation with intervention trials. However, **clinical trials with single small molecules like vitamin E, vitamin C, or β-carotene largely have been disappointing**. (Bjelakovic et al, 2008)

As described earlier, antioxidant defense is multifaceted, thus supplementation with an individual small molecule, unless deficient, likely will have little effect on chronic disease incidence.

A variety of **epidemiological studies** have suggested that intake of lycopene-containing foods, as well as blood lycopene concentrations, are inversely related to incidence of cardiovascular disease and prostate cancer. (Canene-Adams et al, 2005) (Petr, Erdman, 2005) (Voutilainen et al, 2006)

But, these studies have proven nothing, other than that they are highly unreliable.

A 2004 meta-analysis examined the relationship between lycopene/tomato intake and the risk of prostate cancer. The authors found that serum lycopene, lycopene intake, and cooked tomato intake, but not raw tomato intake were associated with a significant decrease in prostate cancer risk. **A number of studies were not included in the analysis, or were published after the meta-analysis**.

Some of these studies report evidence for decreased prostate cancer risk with increased lycopene/tomato exposure. (Comstock et al, 1991)

(Le Marchand et al, 1991) (Schuman et al, 1982) (Goodman et al, 2003) (Wu et al, 2004) (Jian et al, 2005) (McCann et al, 2005) (Zhang et al, 2007) (Sanderson et al, 2004)

Whereas, **some show little to no effect.** (Hayes et al, 1999) (Sonada et al, 2004) (Bosetti et al, 2004) (Kirsh et al, 2006) (Chang et al, 2005) (Peters et al, 2007) (Key et al, 2007) (Pourmand et al, 2007)

There have been 12 small clinical trials investigating the potential impact of lycopene or tomato consumption on prostate cancer risk/progression. These have mostly been in patients; with prostate cancer scheduled for a prostatectomy, with benign prostatic hyperplasia, or at high-risk of developing prostate cancer.

Almost all of these have reported prostate specific antigen (PSA) response (decreased concentration, decreased velocity, increased stabilization) **as an outcome related to disease progression or prostate health.**

Overall, **the majority of these trials have found evidence of improved PSA response with lycopene or tomato consumption, whereas a few have not.** It is important that **these trials be viewed in the context of their small size and general lack of an appropriate control group**.

Lycopene was shown to be 2 and 10-fold more efficient at quenching singlet oxygen than β-carotene and α-tocopherol, respectively, *in vitro*.

But given the substantially higher α-tocopherol content in serum, LDL, and human tissues, even if α-tocopherol has a 10-fold lower antioxidant potential, **it seems unlikely that lycopene plays a meaningful a role as a fellow fat-soluble antioxidant.** (Di Mascio et al, 1989)

Apoptosis is controlled through many tightly-regulated steps which may be modified by dietary intervention. **One human and six animal studies suggest that lycopene induces apoptosis of cancer cells, whereas one human study found no effect.** (Kucuk et al, 2001)

In contrast, **in a mouse emphysema model lycopene decreased the apoptosis rate.** (Kasagi et al, 2006)

The little *in vivo* evidence available suggests that lycopene induces apoptosis in cancer cells.

Overall the available evidence suggests that short-term lycopene feeding may decrease androgen concentrations or signaling. A few studies have also investigated the effects of lycopene consumption on serum estrogen concentrations. **All three *in vivo* human studies identified suggest that lycopene decreases estrogenic activity.** (Cui et al, 2008) (Murtaugh et al, 2004) (Gaudet et al, 2004)

The evidence is mildly suggestive that lycopene may lower estrogen concentrations and/or activity.

Conclusions

There is little *in vivo* data on this topic, therefore we conclude that there is insufficient evidence to support that lycopene decreases CRP.

There is a lack of evidence to suggest that lycopene limits atherosclerosis by decreasing cell surface adhesion molecule expression or intima-media thickness.

We conclude that there is limited experimental support for the "antioxidant hypothesis" as a major mechanism of lycopene's *in vivo* action.

The potential role of lycopene for prostate cancer

The prevention and therapy of prostate cancer: from molecular mechanisms to clinical evidence.

Abstract

Lycopene is a phytochemical that belongs to a group of pigments known as carotenoids. It is red, lipophilic and naturally occurring in many fruits and vegetables, with tomatoes and tomato-based products containing the highest concentrations of bioavailable lycopene. Several epidemiological studies have linked increased lycopene consumption with decreased prostate cancer risk. These findings are supported by in vitro and in vivo experiments showing that lycopene not only enhances the antioxidant response of prostate cells, but that it is even able to inhibit proliferation, induce apoptosis and decrease the metastatic capacity of prostate cancer cells. However, **there is still no clearly proven clinical evidence supporting** the use of lycopene in the prevention or treatment of prostate cancer, due to the only limited number of published randomized clinical trials and the varying quality of existing studies. (Holzapfel et al, 2013)

Effect of Lycopene on Oxidative Stress: Meta-analysis of RCTs

Lycopene supplementation significantly decreases the DNA tail length, as determined using comet assays, with a mean difference (MD) of 6.27 between the lycopene intervention groups and the control groups. Lycopene supplementation does not significantly prolong the lag time of low-density lipoprotein (MD) 3.76. Lycopene possibly alleviates oxidative stress; however, biomarker research for oxidative stress needs be more consistent with the outcomes in lycopene intervention trials for disease prevention.

Oxidative status is assessed in terms of the overall oxidative/reductive potency of a given specimen (e.g., blood or urine) or the susceptibility of various oxidizable components to ex vivo peroxidation.

Lycopene is a potentially powerful antioxidant because of its conjugated double bonds. In vitro evidence suggests that lycopene protects lipoproteins and vascular cells from oxidation, but in vivo evidence is limited.

In 2000, the panel on Dietary Reference Intake evaluated the potential health effects of β-carotene and other carotenoids and concluded that no convincing evidence indicates that substantially increasing the carotenoid intake above current levels significantly affects the antioxidant status; however, lycopene was not specifically addressed.

Considering that lycopene metabolism has not been fully elucidated and antioxidative nutrients interact with each other during gastrointestinal absorption and metabolism, the function of lycopene in vivo possibly differs from that in vitro.

Clinical outcomes

The clinical outcomes assessed in these trials were also analyzed. Clinical outcomes were evaluated in eight trials:

- Lipid profile: No significant differences were found.

- Prostate cancer-related pathologic status: In the trial by Kucuk et al., the pathologic stage of prostate cancer in the lycopene intervention group was less advanced and had lower PSA. **In the trial by Talvas et al., the PSA levels in the healthy men did not change after lycopene intervention**. (Talvas et al, 2010) (Talvas J. Caris-Veyrat C. Guy L, et al. Differential effects of lycopene consumed in tomato paste and lycopene in the form of a purified extract on target genes of cancer prostatic cells. Am J Clin Nutr. 2010;91:1716–1724)

- Inflammatory/immune factors: IL-4 production was reduced by lycopene intervention, TNF-α production was reduced by lycopene intervention, and IgG increased after lycopene intervention.

- Bone resorption marker (NTx): NTx was reduced after lycopene intervention.

- Endothelial cell function: An increase in reactive hyperemia peripheral arterial tonometry (RH-PAT) index from baseline, whereas high-sensitive C-reactive protein (hs-CRP), systolic blood pressure, soluble intercellular adhesion molecule-1 (sICAM-1), and soluble vascular cell adhesion molecule-1 (sVCAM-1) were significantly decreased in the 15 mg/d group.

The present study is the first systematic review of the antioxidative effects of lycopene, in which all available RCTs on the subject were pooled. This review included 13 RCTs, which vary in participant characteristics, formulations, and intervention measures of lycopene, parameters of oxidative stress, and study duration.

Pooling the results of the three trials revealed no statistically significant difference in the LDL lag time between the lycopene treatment group and the controlled group. (Jinyao et al, 2013)

Several factors contributed to the conflicting results of antioxidative activity studies. The null results might have resulted from the very low basal oxidative damage among the young healthy subjects who participated in several studies. Thus, **basal variations are likely negligible and have little biological significance**.

Epidemiologic evidence and dietary intervention studies have associated tomato and lycopene with lower incidence rates of cardiovascular diseases and cancers. However, **the effect of lycopene supplementation remains unconfirmed.**

Tomatoes contain significant amounts of β-carotene, vitamin C, folate, and potassium. Thus, studies on the health benefits of tomatoes should consider other bioactive compounds that could contribute to the beneficial effects investigated.

The contrasting findings on the particular oxidative stress parameters in chronic diseases highlight the importance of validating and standardizing biomarkers for oxidative stress.

We were unable to confirm whether lycopene has different antioxidative effects among subjects with variable physiologic states, or whether lycopene may act differently in short-term versus long-term application. The included trials used variable methods to measure oxidative stress, which caused incomparability across studies.

Given the current evidence, the supposition that lycopene is efficient as an antioxidant *in vivo* needs further examination.

Therefore, until further research establishes significant health benefits for lycopene supplementation in humans, it should be concluded that the **consumption of natural carotenoid-rich fruits and vegetables is preferential to purified lycopene supplementation.** (Jinyao et al, 2013)

Antioxidant supplement effects on heart disease: Meta-analysis of RCTs

Abstract

OBJECTIVE:

To assess the efficacy of vitamin and antioxidant supplements in the prevention of cardiovascular diseases.

DESIGN:

Meta-analysis of randomized controlled trials.

DATA SOURCES AND STUDY SELECTION:

PubMed, EMBASE, the Cochrane Library, Scopus, CINAHL, and ClinicalTrials.gov searched in June and November 2012. Two authors independently reviewed and selected eligible randomized controlled trials, based on predetermined selection criteria.

RESULTS:

Out of 2240 articles retrieved from databases and relevant bibliographies, **50 randomized controlled trials with 294,478 participants** (156,663 in intervention groups and 137,815 in control groups) were included in the final analyses. **In a fixed effect meta-analysis of the 50 trials, supplementation with vitamins and antioxidants was not associated with reductions in the risk of major cardiovascular events.** (Myung et al, 2013)

Overall, there was no beneficial effect of these supplements in the subgroup meta-analyses by type of prevention, type of vitamins and antioxidants, type of cardiovascular outcomes, study design, methodological quality, duration of treatment, funding source, provider of supplements, type of control, number of participants in each trial, and supplements given singly or in combination with other supplements.

Among the subgroup meta-analyses by type of cardiovascular outcomes, *vitamin and antioxidant supplementation was associated with a marginally increased risk of angina pectoris*, while low dose vitamin B(6) supplementation was associated with a slightly decreased risk of major cardiovascular events.

Those beneficial or harmful effects disappeared in subgroup meta-analysis of high quality randomized controlled trials within each category. Also, even though supplementation with vitamin B(6) was associated with a decreased risk of cardiovascular death in high quality trials, and vitamin E supplementation with a decreased risk of myocardial infarction, those beneficial effects were seen only in randomized controlled trials in which the supplements were supplied by the pharmaceutical industry.

CONCLUSION: There is no evidence to support the use of vitamin and antioxidant supplements for prevention of cardiovascular diseases. (Myung et al, 2013)

Effect of antioxidant vitamins on cardiovascular outcomes: Meta-analysis of RCTs

Abstract

BACKGROUND:

Antioxidant vitamin (vitamin E, beta-carotene, and vitamin C) are widely used for preventing major cardiovascular outcomes. However, the effect of antioxidant vitamin on cardiovascular events remains unclear.

METHODOLOGY AND PRINCIPAL FINDINGS:

We searched PubMed, EmBase, the Cochrane Central Register of Controlled Trials, and the proceedings of major conferences for relevant literature. Eligible studies were randomized controlled trials that reported on the effects of antioxidant vitamin on cardiovascular outcomes as compared to placebo. Outcomes analyzed were major cardiovascular events, myocardial infarction, stroke, cardiac death, total death, and any possible adverse events. We used the I(2) statistic to measure heterogeneity between trials and calculated risk estimates for cardiovascular outcomes with random-effect meta-analysis. Independent extraction was performed by two reviewers and consensus was reached. Of 293 identified studies, **we included 15 trials reporting data on 188,209 participants.** These studies reported 12749 major cardiovascular events, 6699 myocardial infarction, 3749 strokes, 14122 total death, and 5980 cardiac deaths. Overall, antioxidant vitamin supplementation as compared to placebo had no effect on major cardiovascular events (RR, 1.00; 95%CI, 0.96-1.03), myocardial infarction (RR, 0.98; 95%CI, 0.92-1.04), stroke (RR, 0.99; 95%CI, 0.93-1.05), total death (RR, 1.03; 95%CI, 0.98-1.07), cardiac death (RR, 1.02; 95%CI, 0.97-1.07), revascularization (RR, 1.00; 95%CI, 0.95-1.05), total CHD (RR, 0.96; 95%CI, 0.87-1.05), angina (RR, 0.98; 95%CI, 0.90-1.07), and congestive heart failure (RR, 1.07; 95%CI, 0.96 to 1.19).

CONCLUSION/SIGNIFICANCE

Antioxidant vitamin supplementation has no effect on the incidence of major cardiovascular events, myocardial infarction, stroke, total death, cardiac death, revascularization, total CHD, angina and congestive heart failure. (Ye, Yuan, 2013)

Prof Randolph M Howes MD,PhD

Effect of antioxidant vitamins in myocardial infarction

Abstract

Acute myocardial infarction (AMI) is the leading cause of mortality worldwide. Major advances in the treatment of acute coronary syndromes and myocardial infarction, using cardiologic interventions, such as thrombolysis or percutaneous coronary angioplasty (PCA) have improved the clinical outcome of patients. Nevertheless, as a consequence of these procedures, the ischemic zone is reperfused, giving rise to a lethal reperfusion event accompanied by increased production of reactive oxygen species (oxidative stress). These reactive species attack biomolecules such as lipids, DNA, and proteins enhancing the previously established tissue damage, as well as triggering cell death pathways. Studies on animal models of AMI suggest that lethal reperfusion accounts for up to 50% of the final size of a myocardial infarct, a part of the damage likely to be prevented. **Although a number of strategies have been aimed at to ameliorate lethal reperfusion injury, up to date the beneficial effects in clinical settings have been disappointing [for antioxidant vitamins].** (Rodrigo et al, 2013)

Tomatoes and lycopene in prevention and therapy

Is there an evidence for prostate diseases?

Abstract

Tomatoes are discussed to have an important role in the prevention of and therapy for prostate cancer (PCA). Whether or not they are also useful in the primary and secondary prevention of benign prostate hyperplasia (BPH) is not clear. Whereas **epidemiological studies on BPH prevention provide no evidence for a preventive potential of tomatoes and tomato products**, the majority of interventional trials points to an increased DNA resistance against oxidative-induced damage. Even though their effect on a surrogate marker of the IGF pathway cannot be evaluated so far due to insufficient data, the consumption of tomatoes and tomato products may probably protect from PCA--at least when considering low-grade PCA. Thus, regular consumption of these foods can be recommended for the prevention of PCA. **The intake of isolated lycopene does**

not protect from the development of prostate cancer (PCA).
(Ellinger et al, 2009)

Lycopene may block killing of cancer cells

Lycopene supplementation prevents reactive oxygen species mediated apoptosis in Sertoli cells of adult albino rats exposed to polychlorinated biphenyls.

Abstract

Sertoli cell proliferation is attenuated before attaining puberty and the number is fixed in adult testes. Sertoli cells determine both testis size and daily sperm production by providing physical and metabolic support to spermatogenic cells. Polychlorinated biphenyls (PCBs) exposure disrupts functions of Sertoli cells causing infertility with decreased sperm count. On the other hand, lycopene is improving sperm count and motility by reducing oxidative stress in humans and animals. Hence we hypothesized that PCBs-induced infertility might be due to Sertoli cell apoptosis mediated by oxidative stress and lycopene might prevent PCBs-induced apoptosis by acting against oxidative stress. To test this hypothesis, animals were treated with vehicle control, lycopene, PCBs and PCBs + lycopene for 30 days. After the experimental period, the testes and cauda epididymidis were removed for isolation of Sertoli cells and sperm, respectively. We observed increased levels of oxidative stress markers (H2O2 and LPO) levels, increased expression of apoptotic molecules (caspase-8, Bad, Bid, Bax, cytochrome C and caspase-3), decreased anti-apoptotic (Bcl2) molecule and elevated apoptotic marker activity (caspase-3) in Sertoli cells of PCBs-exposed animals. These results were associated with decreased sperm count and motility in PCBs exposed animals. On the other hand, lycopene prevented the elevation of Sertoli cellular apoptotic parameters and prevented the reduction of sperm parameters (count and motility). The data confirmed that **lycopene as an antioxidant scavenged reactive oxygen substances, prevented apoptosis,** maintained normal function in Sertoli cells and helped to provide physical and metabolic support for sperm production, thereby treating infertility in men. (Krishnamoorthy et al, 2013)

Both chemotherapy and radiation therapy kill cancer cells by prooxidant induced apoptosis. Thus, prooxidants can be tumoricidal and it appears that **lycopene can block the cancer killing ability of chemo and radiation therapy.**

Lycopene and fish oil effect on prostate cancer: an RCT

Gene expression and biological pathways in tissue of men with prostate cancer in a randomized clinical trial of lycopene and fish oil supplementation.

Abstract

BACKGROUND:

Studies suggest that micronutrients may modify the risk or delay progression of prostate cancer; however, the molecular mechanisms involved are poorly understood. We examined the effects of lycopene and fish oil on prostate gene expression in a double-blind placebo-controlled randomized clinical trial.

METHODS:

Eighty-four men with low risk prostate cancer were stratified based on self-reported dietary consumption of fish and tomatoes and then randomly assigned to a 3-month intervention of lycopene (n=29) or fish oil (n=27) supplementation or placebo (n=28). Gene expression in morphologically normal prostate tissue was studied at baseline and at 3 months via cDNA microarray analysis. Differential gene expression and pathway analyses were performed to identify genes and pathways modulated by these micronutrients.

RESULTS

Global gene expression analysis revealed no significant individual genes that were associated with high intake of fish or tomato at baseline or after 3 months of supplementation with lycopene or fish oil.

CONCLUSIONS:

We did not detect significant individual genes associated with dietary intake and supplementation of lycopene and fish oil. (Magbanua et al, 2011) 1)

Effect of tomato paste on genes of prostate cancer cells

Differential effects of lycopene consumed in tomato paste and lycopene in the form of a purified extract on target genes of cancer prostatic cells.

Abstract

BACKGROUND:

Prospective studies indicate that tomato consumers are protected against prostate cancer. Lycopene has been hypothesized to be responsible for tomato health benefits.

OBJECTIVE:

Our aim was to differentiate the effects of tomato matrix from those of lycopene by using lycopene-rich red tomatoes, lycopene-free yellow tomatoes, and purified lycopene.

DESIGN:

Thirty healthy men (aged 50-70 y old) were randomly assigned to 2 groups after a 2-wk washout period. In a crossover design, each group consumed yellow and red tomato paste (200 g/d, which provided 0 and 16 mg lycopene, respectively) as part of their regular diet for 1 wk separated by 2 wk of washout. Then, in a parallel design, the first group underwent supplementation with purified lycopene (16 mg/d) for 1 wk, whereas the second group received a placebo. Sera collected before and after the interventions were incubated with lymph node cancer prostate cells to measure the expression of 45 target genes.

RESULTS:

Circulating lycopene concentration increased only after consumption of red tomato paste and purified lycopene.

Lipid profile, antioxidant status, prostate-specific antigen, and insulin-like growth factor 1 were not modified by consumption of tomato pastes and lycopene. We observed significant up-regulation of IGFBP-3 and Bax: Bcl-2 ratio and down-regulation of cyclin-D1, p53, and Nrf-2 after cell incubation with sera from men who consumed red tomato paste when compared with sera collected after the first washout period, with intermediate values for yellow tomato paste consumption. Cell incubation with sera from men who consumed purified lycopene led to significant up-regulation of IGFBP-3, c-fos, and uPAR compared with sera collected after placebo consumption.

CONCLUSION: Dietary lycopene can affect gene expression whether or not it is included in its food matrix. This trial was registered by the French Health Ministry at http://www.sante-sports.gouv.fr as 2006-A00396-45. (Talvas et al, 2010)

Effect of garlic and tomato on Ehrlich ascites tumors

Long-Term Treatment with Aqueous Garlic and/or Tomato Suspensions Decreases Ehrlich Ascites Tumors

We evaluated the preventive and therapeutic effects of aqueous suspensions of garlic, tomato, and garlic + tomato in the development of experimental Ehrlich tumors in mice. The aqueous suspensions (2%) were administered over a short term for 30 days before tumor inoculation and 12 days afterward, and suspensions at 6% were administered for 180 days before inoculation and for 12 days afterward. The volume, number, and characteristics of the tumor cells and AgNOR counts were determined to compare the different treatments. Aqueous 6% suspensions of garlic, tomato, and garlic + tomato given over the long term significantly reduced tumor growth but when given over the short term, they did not alter tumor growth.

Cancer is a disease of complex etiology. It is now recognized that a great majority of human cancers, perhaps as many as 80–90%, are attributable to environmental factors.

The prevention of cancer through the ingestion of vegetables and fruits has been suggested in human epidemiologic studies. The induction of apoptosis is currently recognized as a useful strategy to treat and prevent cancer, and a large number of natural dietary constituents have been reported to induce apoptosis in malignant cells.

These findings are consistent with the observation that **high consumption of fruits and vegetables is associated with reduced risk of various cancers; in particular, tomato and garlic are recognized to possess a wide range of beneficial effects**.

Garlic (bulb of *Allium sativum*), a common plant used as a food item as well as a medicinal herb in many countries of the world, is one of the most ancient plants reputed to have cancerostatic effects, as well as antiviral, antifungal, and antibacterial activities, and the ability to lower blood lipid levels and blood pressure.

Garlic contains at least thirty-three sulfur compounds, several enzymes, and seventeen amino acids. Additional constituents of intact garlic include steroidal glycosides and lectins. The sulfur compounds are responsible for garlic's pungent odor and many of its medicinal effects. The anticarcinogenic properties of garlic have been indicated in several studies.

Beneficial effects of tomato (*Lycopersicon esculentum*) were observed against cancer of the pancreas, colon, rectum, esophagus, and breast. Lycopene, which is found in tomato-based products, belongs to the carotenoid family, a group of more than 1000 plant and animal pigments involved in photosynthesis and photoprotection. Lycopene may be important in preventing prostate cancer.

Transplantable experimental tumors have been used in studies of physical, chemical, viral, and hormonal carcinogenesis. Ehrlich tumor is a transplantable neoplasm from a malign epithelium, such as mammary adenocarcinoma in female mice. When inoculated intraperitoneally, the tumor grows in an ascitic form.

In this study, we compared the effects of aqueous garlic and/or tomato suspensions administered over a short and long term on the prevention and treatment of experimental Ehrlich ascites tumors in mice.

In the first experiment, when treating the animals for a short period (30 days before inoculation and 12 days after inoculation), we observed that **tumor growth was the same in all experimental groups, with no statistically significant differences between animals treated with aqueous suspensions of garlic, tomato, or garlic + tomato relative to the control**.

We observed the mean volume of ascites tumors, solid tumor mass, number of cells per mL, and the total number of tumor cells but **found no significant differences between the groups**.

However, in the second experiment, we observed that the groups administered aqueous suspensions of garlic and garlic + tomato at 6% over the long term (180 days before tumor inoculation and 12 days after inoculation) showed significantly reduced tumor growth.

The beneficial anticarcinogenic and immunomodulatory effects of the agents in garlic, that is, water- and lipid-soluble allyl sulfides, can influence a number of molecular events involved in cancer, such as inhibiting mutagenesis, blocking carcinogen DNA adduct formation, scavenging free radicals, and blocking cell proliferation, differentiation, and angiogenesis.

Carotenoids found in tomatoes are fat-soluble pigments responsible for the yellow, orange, and red colors in many fruits and vegetables. Lycopene has the strongest antioxidant properties of the carotenoids, and higher intake has been associated with a reduced risk of many cancer types, including prostate, lung, and stomach. Recent work in cancer cell lines and animal models has demonstrated that lycopene can reduce the transcription of steroid-related genes, insulin-like growth factor-1 expression, and inflammatory signals, suggesting that these pathways may account, in part, for the inverse association between lycopene and the risk of some cancers.

We observed that **the bioactive compounds in garlic and/or tomato administered for a short period did not prevent or reduce the development of experimental Ehrlich ascites tumors in BALB/c mice**.

However, **when we increased the concentration of the aqueous garlic and/or tomato suspension and administered the solution for a long period (for 6 months), the anticancer effects of garlic and/or tomato were observed because the growth of the tumor was lower in treated than in untreated animals**.

Ehrlich tumors are rapidly growing carcinomas with aggressive behavior. They are able to grow in nearly all mouse strains, which suggests that the recognition and immune responses to these tumors are independent of the MHC. This characteristic suggests that controlling an Ehrlich tumor is more related to innate immunity, especially the inflammatory response, than to T cell responses.

The Ehrlich ascites tumor implantation induces per se a local inflammatory reaction, with increasing vascular permeability, which results in the formation of an intense edema and progressive ascites fluid and cellular migration.

In the same way, it is possible that garlic and onion exert their anti-carcinogen actions indirectly by different mechanisms, such as through inhibition of lipoxygenase and cyclooxygenase activities (an anti-inflammatory effect).
(Bom et al, 2014)

Lycopene and male infertility: do we know enough?

The following was excerpted or modified from: (Pakrashi, Oihninger, 2014)

There has been a recent renewed interest in the medical treatment of male subfertility. Although, intracytoplasmic sperm injection can surmount many of the reproductive challenges imposed upon couples struggling with male infertility, it remains an invasive and expensive treatment modality.

Infections and inflammation, smoking, environmental exposure to toxins and heat, anatomic abnormalities such as varicocele and cryptorchidism, **may** all result in oxidative stress. (Ko, Sabanegh, 2014)

Oxidative stress leads to the production of reactive oxygen species (ROS, EMODs). Antioxidants present in seminal plasma and spermatozoa serve to maintain a balance and protect against damage caused by ROS. Excessive amounts of ROS can cause structural damage to the sperm deoxyribonucleic acid, reduce motility and damage the sperm membrane, leading to abnormal semen parameters and possibly, infertility. (Ross et al, 2010)

Thus, the use of antioxidant therapy has garnered attention in the treatment of reversible causes of male infertility. In this issue of the journal, Durairajanayagam et al. present an exhaustive review of animal and human data associating a lycopene-enriched diet with an improvement in markers of oxidative stress in semen and other parameters. The authors indicate the potential for lycopene supplementation in idiopathic male infertility. (Durairajanayagam et al, 2014)

Lycopene, a lipid soluble carotenoid found in tomato-rich diets, is a powerful scavenger of free radicals preventing lipid peroxidation.

Data suggest the beneficial effect of lycopene-rich diets on chronic disease states by upregulating gap-junction communication and modulation of growth factors.

A recent publication suggested the protective effect of lycopene against polychlorinated biphenyl induced epididymal toxicity in a rat model. (Raj et al, 2014)

To study differences in the nutrient intake of men with normal semen parameters and those with low sperm numbers, motility or morphology, Mendiola *et al.* examined specific nutrient intake of men attending infertility clinics in Spain. The authors demonstrated a positive association between lycopene intake and semen quality. (Mendiola et al, 2010)

The present data linking lycopene to an improvement in semen parameters is primarily observational, with small sample sizes under investigation. The limitations conferred by bias and confounding in current literature makes it difficult to look beyond an association, despite biological plausibility.

Supplementation of diet with antioxidants has been studied in other areas of medicine. Sommer *et al.* discuss the example of Vitamins E and C, which have been associated with a reduced risk of cataract formation in observational studies. **The seemingly beneficial effect of a reduction of cataract formation with Vitamin C or E supplementation was not replicated in a well-designed randomized controlled trial.** (Sommer, Vyas, 2012)

Similarly, epidemiologic studies suggest a beneficial effect of lycopene on cardiovascular health. However, **in a randomized controlled trial, lycopene supplementation in moderately overweight, disease-free, middle aged adults (an appropriate target population for lycopene supplementation in clinical practice) showed no significant changes in markers of cardiovascular disease. These findings do not justify potential health claims that lycopene supplementation has a cardioprotective effect.** (Thies et al, 2012)

The review by Durairajanayagam *et al.* underscores the need for prospective and randomized controlled trials in male subfertility treated with lycopene as a nutritional supplement. This is because **observational studies cannot establish cause and effect.**

Clinical associations do not always hold up when subjected to the rigors of a randomized controlled trial. Until then, we must tread cautiously. (Pakrashi, Oihninger, 2014)

A global clinical view on vitamin A and carotenoids
(Sommer, Vyas, 2012)

Abstract

The clinical importance of vitamin A as an essential nutrient has become increasingly clear. Adequate vitamin A is required for normal organogenesis, immune competence, tissue differentiation, and the visual cycle. Deficiency, which is widespread throughout the developing world, is responsible for a million or more instances of unnecessary death and blindness each year. β-Carotene is an important, but insufficient, source of vitamin A among poor populations, which accounts for the widespread nature of vitamin A deficiency.

It has only recently become apparent that the bioconversion of traditional dietary sources of β-carotene to vitamin A is much less efficient than previously supposed.

The other major carotenoids, **particularly lycopene**, lutein, and zeaxanthin, have been found to have important biological properties, including antioxidant and photoprotective activity, and high intake has been linked in observational studies with reduced risk of a number of chronic diseases.

But, **to date, 2012, no clinical trials have proven the clinical value of ingested carotenoids individually or in combination, in either physiologic or pharmacologic doses, with the exception of the provitamin A activity of carotene**.

Indeed, several trials have suggested an increased risk of lung cancer among high-risk individuals (smokers and asbestos workers) who were given high doses of β-carotene alone or in combination with other antioxidants. **Much more evidence is needed before commonly encountered claims of the value of ingesting high doses of nonprovitamin A carotenoids are validated. RMH Note: Please remember that lycopene is not converted into vitamin A.**

A radical approach includes genetically bioengineered crops, such as "golden rice," which contains highly bioavailable β-carotene in a food in which it does not naturally occur, or those that offer a dramatic increase in β-carotene, such as tomatoes.

Prof Randolph M Howes MD,PhD

Carotenoids have become a major area of scientific inquiry and big business, with sales projected to reach $1.2 billion by 2015.

Adequate intake of carotenoids is purportedly important for the prevention of all manner of disease. Yet, whereas supplies of vegetables and fruit vary dramatically around the world, **there is little clinical evidence that any sizeable population consumes inadequate amounts for normal physiologic function**. In other words, **these are not "essential nutrients" in the traditional sense, and, as matters now stand, their "deficiency" does not result in clinically recognizable disease**. Of course, we must remain open to the possibility that such deficiency disease or diseases might exist: only relatively recently was vitamin A deficiency definitively recognized to influence immune competence and increase infectious morbidity and mortality, despite previous suspicions that this might be the case. Until such time as true, carotenoid "deficiency"–related clinical entities are discovered, the only natural physiologic role recognized to be important is that of the provitamin A activity of carotenes, especially β-carotene.

More worrisome still are the outcomes of several large, particularly well-conducted randomized clinical trials. Randomized trials are the "gold standard" for proving the value of reversing a "deficiency" or of increasing the intake of a particular substance in pharmaceutical amounts. These have failed to find any consistent reduction in the incidence of cancers or cancer deaths, or of cardiovascular disease, among individuals randomly assigned to receive β-carotene, with or without α-tocopherol or retinol and the Alpha-Tocopherol, Beta Carotene Cancer Prevention Study Group.
(Hennekens et al, 1996)

Worse still, in 2 of these trials, which specifically enrolled participants at high risk of lung cancer (smokers and/or asbestos workers) the active agents appeared to increase the risk of developing lung cancer. Subsequent systematic reviews of the literature confirm the potential for increased cancer risks from β-carotene supplementation.

Why these apparently conflicting clinical and epidemiologic results? The most obvious reason is that purely observational studies are prone to suffer from bias. People who eat the most salad are likely to differ in many other ways from those who eat much less. Whereas these studies purportedly "adjust" for other differences in lifestyle and known risks, they cannot "adjust" for them all, nor necessarily for the most important. No study can collect data on every potentially important variable, and the most important variables may not even be known. Even if frequent consumption of salad, by itself, reduces the risk of certain diseases, salads contain an enormous number of different compounds, not just β-carotene or carotenoids in general.

Clearly, new and very different research designs are needed to begin to dissect out which dietary carotenoids (or combinations of carotenoids) are important for promoting health and preventing disease, if indeed there are diseases that increased carotenoid intake can help to prevent. The fact that lutein and zeaxanthin are highly concentrated in the macula strongly suggests that they might play a vital physiologic role.

But, we must remain mindful that other nutrients thought to have antioxidant qualities, such as vitamins E and C for example, and that are associated in observational studies with a reduced risk of cataract formation in humans have failed to show any such benefit when tested in tightly controlled randomized trials.

Until definitive clinical evidence becomes available, we can only conclude that humans accumulate a variety of carotenoids, but their importance and roles remain uncertain. The only well-established pathophysiologic consequence of dietary carotenoid "deficiency" remains the provitamin A activity of carotene, especially β-carotene.

SECTION THREE

COENZYME Q; UBIQUINONE
CoQ10 ANTIOXIDANT

Summary of factoids on CoQ10 antioxidants

Overall CoQ10 facts

- Coenzyme Q10 (CoQ10) is an antioxidant found in every cell in the body and aids in energy production.

- **It is also known as Q10, vitamin Q10, ubiquinone, or ubidecarenone.**

- **CoQ10 isn't actually vitamin, as the body produces its own supply**.

- **A number of prescription medicines (beta-blockers, statins and some oral anti-diabetes drugs) can lower CoQ10 levels in the body**.

- **Since no one company can patent CoQ10, no entity is motivated to fund expensive clinical trials.**

- It is claimed to support cardiovascular health and prevent high blood pressure.

Positive

- **CoQ protected endothelial cells from Aβ-induced injury at physiological concentrations in human plasma after oral CoQ supplementation and thus could be a promising molecule to protect endothelial cells against amyloid angiopathy**. However, this was a totally in vitro study. (Duran-Prado et al, 2014)

- This study suggest that **coenzyme Q10 exert beneficial effects on the lipid profile, atherogenic index, and liver enzymes activity in alloxan-induced type 1 diabetic rats.** (Ahmadvand, Ghaseme-Dehnoo, 2014)

- **Supplementation of statin-treated patients with CoQ10 resulted in a decrease in the symptoms of statin-associated myopathy (SAM), both in absolute numbers and intensity**. Additional selenium supplementation was not associated with any statistically significant decrease of SAM. **However, it is not possible to draw any definite conclusions**, even though this study was carried out in double-blind fashion, because **it involved a small number of patients**. (Fedacko et al, 2013)

Negative

- **Research is not consistent and the American Heart Association does not recommend CoQ10 for people with congestive heart failure**.

- **Millions took antioxidant vitamins for years thinking that they were heart healthy, when evidence eventually showed they are at best, useless, and at worst, harmful.**

- **Human studies have shot down the theory that extra CoQ10 can boost your energy or endurance or help treat gum disease.** (Watts, 1995)

- **Animal studies have suggested that CoQ10 might combat brain deterioration in Alzheimer's patients, but results in humans are disappointing so far.**

- **The Mayo Clinic website lists as unclear the use of CoQ10 with antiaging, asthma, breast cancer, eye health, cataracts, chemotherapy side effects, chest pain, chronic fatigue syndrome, cocaine dependence, coronary heart disease, cystic fibrosis, dry mouth, exercise performance, fibromyalgia, gum disease, hearing loss, heart attack, chronic myocardial** disease, heart disease prevention, heart muscle injury, high cholesterol, **HIV/AIDS**, hypertriglyceridemia, immune enhancement, infant development/neonatal care, kidney failure, male infertility, migraine, mitochondrial diseases, mitral valve prolapse, movement disorders, muscle weakness, muscular dystrophies, myelodysplastic syndrome, nerve pain, Parkinson's disease, Peyronie's disease, pre-eclampsia, prostate cancer, psoriasis, recovery from surgery, ringing in the ears and weight loss.

- **CoQ10 has not been shown definitely to relieve heart failure symptoms.** Only some of the studies of coenzyme Q10 showed that it helps heart failure symptoms. (Med Ltr, 2006) (Coenzyme Q10 (2006). Medical Letter on Drugs and Therapeutics, 48(1229): 19–20)

- **The National Cancer Institute (NCI) rates the strength of the evidence for CoQ10 and cancer (secondary treatment) as weak.** (NCI, 2012)

- **Research does not support a helpful effect of CoQ10 in periodontal (gum) disease, muscular dystrophy, or exercise recovery.** (WebMD.com)

- **Pooled analysis suggests that the use of coenzyme Q10 has no clear effect on left ventricular ejection fraction or exercise capacity. No conclusions can be drawn on the benefits or harms of coenzyme Q10 in heart failure at this time (2014). Their results are inconclusive.** (Madmani et al, 2014)

- **For diastolic blood pressure we performed a random-effects meta-analysis, which showed no evidence of effect of CoQ10 supplementation. The trial showed no evidence of effect of CoQ10 supplementation on total cholesterol, high-density lipoprotein (HDL)-cholesterol or triglycerides.**

- Of the four trials that investigated CoQ10 supplementation in patients on statin therapy, **three of them showed that simultaneous administration of CoQ10 did not significantly influence lipid levels or systolic blood pressure levels** between the two groups. *The fourth trial showed a significant increase in the change in total and low-density lipoprotein (LDL)-cholesterol at three months across the four arms of the trial* (α-tocopherol, CoQ10, CoQ10 + α-tocopherol and placebo). **There was no significant difference in the change in HDL-cholesterol and triglycerides after three months between the four arms of the trial.** (Flowers et al, 2014)

- *CoQ levels were similar among pulmonary arterial hypertension (PAH) and control individuals, and increased in all subjects with CoQ supplementation.* **Metabolic and redox parameters, including lactate, pyruvate and reduced or oxidized glutathione, did not change in PAH patients with CoQ.** (Sharp et al, 2014)

- CoQ(10) treatment increased plasma CoQ(10) levels from 1.1 +/-0.5 to 5.0+/-2.8 micromol/l but had no significant effect on Flow-mediated (FMD, endothelium-dependent) and nitrate-mediated (NMD, smooth muscle-dependent) arterial dilatation or serum LDL-cholesterol levels. We conclude that **dietary supplementation with CoQ(10) decreases ex-vivo LDL oxidizability but has no significant effect on arterial endothelial function in patients with moderate hypercholesterolemia.** (Raitakari et al, 2000)

- **The endothelial function assessed peripherally by nitrate-mediated arterial dilatation was not significantly improved with CoQ10 by using fix-effects model.** (Gao et al, 2011)

- **CoQ-10 has a relaxing effect on blood vessels, it can lower blood pressure levels.** *If taken with a high blood pressure medication, CoQ-10 can cause blood pressure to drop too low.*

- *CoQ-10 can also reduce the effectiveness of blood thinners such as heparin, warfarin, or even aspirin.*

- **CoQ10 rarely causes side effects.** *Occasionally, it causes stomach upset or diarrhea, especially when more than 100 milligrams is taken in a single dose.*

- *CoQ10 can reduce the effect of the blood thinner Coumadin (Warfarin).* (Spigset, 1994) (Landbo, Almdal, 1998)

- **Coenzyme Q10 treatment does not slow the progression of Parkinson's disease (PD). This was the disappointing conclusion of a Phase 3 clinical trial designed to test the disease-modifying potential of the drug.** The results were **published March 24, 2014 in JAMA Neurology. Disease symptoms progressed just as quickly in both CoQ10 groups as in the placebo group. The investigators concluded that CoQ10 showed no evidence of benefit in early Parkinson's Disease patients.**

- In 2007, the National Institute of Neurological Disorders and Stroke Neuroprotection Exploratory Trials (NET-PD) consortium tested 2400 mg CoQ10 in PD patients (see NET-PD, 2007). (NET-PD, 2007) A primary analysis of the results, which relied on historical controls, deemed CoQ10 worthy of moving into a larger trial. **However, a secondary analysis using controls that more closely resembled the treatment group found that continuing with the drug would be futile.** (Snow et al, 2010)

- There were no significant differences between the CoQ10 and placebo arms at 24 weeks for scores (CoQ10's effects on self-reported fatigue, depression, and quality of life (QOL)) on the Profile of Mood States-Fatigue questionnaire, the Functional Assessment of Chronic Illness Therapy-Fatigue tool, the Functional Assessment of Cancer Therapy-Breast Cancer instrument, or the Center for Epidemiologic Studies-Depression scale. **Supplementation with conventional doses of CoQ10 led to sustained increases in plasma CoQ10 levels but did not result in improved self-reported fatigue or QOL after 24 weeks of treatment.** (Lesser et al, 2013)

- **CoQ10 did not produce a greater response than placebo in the treatment of presumed statin-induced myalgias.** (Bookstaver et al, 2012)

- **This study revealed no significant effects of CoQ10 and selenium on statin-induced myopathy (SIM) compared with the placebo.** (Bogsrud et al, 2013)

- **Overall, results of the study demonstrate that children and adolescents with migraine improved over time with multidisciplinary, standardized treatment regardless of supplementation with CoQ10 or placebo. There was no difference in headache outcomes between the CoQ10 and placebo groups at day 224.** (Slater et al, 2011) a randomized in a crossover, double-blind, placebo-controlled, randomized, add-on study.

CoQ10 general information from WebMD

http://www.webmd.com/heart-disease/heart-failure/tc/coenzyme-q10-topic-overview (Accessed 12-23-14)

Coenzyme Q10 (CoQ10) is a substance similar to a vitamin. It is found in every cell of the body. Your body makes CoQ10, and your cells use it to produce energy your body needs for cell growth and maintenance. **It also functions as an antioxidant.**

CoQ10 is naturally present in small amounts in a wide variety of foods, but levels are particularly high in organ meats such as heart, liver, and kidney, as well as beef, soy oil, sardines, mackerel, and peanuts.

Coenzymes help enzymes work to digest food and perform other body processes, and they help protect the heart and skeletal muscles.

CoQ10 is available in the United States as a dietary supplement. **It is also known as Q10, vitamin Q10, ubiquinone, or ubidecarenone.**

Many claims are made about CoQ10. It is said to help heart failure, as well as cancer, muscular dystrophy, and periodontal disease. It is also said to boost energy and speed recovery from exercise. Some people take it to help reduce the effects certain medicines can have on the heart, muscles, and other organs.

If you have heart failure, talk to your doctor before you take any supplement. **There's no strong evidence that vitamins or other supplements can help treat heart failure.** They are used along with medical heart failure treatments, not instead of treatment.

But you may still hear about CoQ10 supplements and heart failure. **CoQ10 has not been shown definitely to relieve heart failure symptoms.** Only some of the studies of coenzyme Q10 showed that it helps heart failure symptoms. (Med Ltr, 2006)

CoQ10 and cancer

In 1961, scientists saw that people with cancer had little CoQ10 in their blood. They found low CoQ10 blood levels in people with myeloma, lymphoma, and cancers of the breast, lung, prostate, pancreas, colon, kidney, and head and neck. Some research has suggested that CoQ10 helps the immune system and may be useful as a secondary treatment for cancer.

- CoQ10 may keep the antitumor drug doxorubicin from hurting the heart.

- Three studies examined the use of CoQ10 along with conventional treatment for cancer. The three studies contained a total of 41 women with breast cancer. In each study, the women improved.

But **the National Cancer Institute (NCI) rates the strength of the evidence for CoQ10 and cancer (secondary treatment) as weak.** (NCI, 2012)

Other claims

Research does not support a helpful effect of CoQ10 in periodontal (gum) disease, muscular dystrophy, or exercise recovery.

Side effects

Taking 100 mg a day or more of CoQ10 has caused mild insomnia in some people. And research has detected elevated levels of liver enzymes in people taking doses of 300 mg per day for long periods of time. Liver toxicity has not been reported.

Other reported side effects include rashes, nausea, upper abdominal pain, dizziness, sensitivity to light, irritability, headache, heartburn, and fatigue.

Medicines for high cholesterol (statins) and medicines that lower blood sugar cause a decrease of CoQ10 levels and reduce the effects of CoQ10 supplements.

CoQ10 can reduce the body's response to the blood thinner (anticoagulant) medicine warfarin (Coumadin) and can decrease insulin requirements in people with diabetes.

The U.S. Food and Drug Administration (FDA) does not regulate dietary supplements in the same way it regulates medicines. **A dietary supplement can be sold with limited or no research on how well it works or on its safety.**

When using dietary supplements, keep in mind the following:

- Like conventional medicines, dietary supplements may cause side effects, trigger allergic reactions, or interact with prescription and nonprescription medicines or other supplements you might be taking. A side effect or interaction with another medicine or supplement may make other health conditions worse. Always tell your doctor or pharmacist about all dietary supplements you are taking.

- The way dietary supplements are manufactured may not be standardized. Because of this, how well they work or any side effects they cause may differ among brands or even within different lots of the same brand. The form of supplement that you buy in health food or grocery stores may not be the same as the form used in research.

- Other than for vitamins and minerals, the long-term effects of most dietary supplements are not known.

This information is produced and provided by the National Cancer Institute (NCI). (Last updated, 2013).

The Mayo Clinic discusses CoQ10

Here are the Mayo Clinic's pie-in-the-sky *unreferenced claims*: (Mayo Clinic. org)

There is some evidence that idebenone, a man-made compound similar to CoQ10, may benefit people with Alzheimer's disease. However, the effect of CoQ10 itself is unclear.

The results for treating ALS is unclear. CoQ10 has been studied for amyotrophic lateral sclerosis (ALS), a disease affecting brain and spinal cord nerve cells that control muscle movement. More research is needed in this area.

CoQ10 may benefit men with Peyronie's disease (abnormal curvature, pain, and scar tissue in the penis) in terms of slowing disease progression and reducing curvature.

Early research suggests that CoQ10 may lower the occurrence of pre-eclampsia (high blood pressure during pregnancy) in women who are at risk.

A combination product containing CoQ10 may improve symptoms of psoriasis, an inflammatory skin condition.

Early research reports that CoQ10 may benefit people who have nerve pain caused by diabetes.

CoQ10 has been studied for myelodysplastic syndrome, a condition in which there is cell damage in the bone marrow. Early evidence suggests that CoQ10 may benefit people who have this condition.

There is mixed evidence in support of CoQ10 or idebenone (a man-made compound similar to CoQ10) for treating muscular dystrophies, diseases in which there is muscle damage or loss.

Early evidence suggests that CoQ10 may be useful in treating symptoms of Friedreich's ataxia, a disease that damages the nervous system.

CoQ10 has been studied for diseases affecting the mitochondria, which are energy-creating components found in every cell in the body. There is promising evidence to support CoQ10 use for conditions such as Kearns-Sayre syndrome, which may cause drooping eyelids and vision problems.

Early research suggests that CoQ10 may help treat symptoms of Prader-Labhart-Willi syndrome, a genetic disorder affecting growth and development.

CoQ10 has been studied for immune enhancement. However, details are lacking.

There is promising evidence to support the use of CoQ10 before heart surgery.

Research suggests that CoQ10 may benefit people who have cardiomyopathy, a weakening or problem with the heart muscle. Levels of CoQ10 may be lower in people with this condition.

CoQ10 may improve blood flow and blood vessel widening in people with diabetes. A combination of CoQ10 and garlic extract may benefit heart health associated with stress.

CoQ10 may have benefits in people with a chronic disease of the heart muscle.

CoQ10 may benefit people who have had a previous heart attack.

Low levels of CoQ10 may be associated with a higher risk of hearing loss.

Early research suggests that CoQ10 levels may be lower in the gum tissue of people with gum disease. There is promising evidence to support CoQ10 for treating gum disease.

Fibromyalgia is a condition in which there is long-term pain and tenderness in the muscles and joints. Early study suggests that people with this disorder may benefit from the use of CoQ10.

Overall, strong evidence is lacking on the use of CoQ10 for improving exercise performance.

CoQ10 may most benefit people who have chronic lung diseases, such as asthma.

Early research suggests that CoQ10 may improve symptoms of dry mouth.

Low levels of CoQ10 have been found in children with cystic fibrosis, a disease that causes mucus buildup in lungs. Combination products containing CoQ10 have been studied. More research on the effects of CoQ10 alone is needed.

CoQ10 used in combination with the cholesterol-lowering drug simvastatin may benefit people who have coronary heart disease. CoQ10 may also help reduce inflammation in those with this condition.

Early research shows that CoQ10 may improve symptoms of chronic fatigue syndrome.

CoQ10 levels may help predict the risk of skin cancer progression. One study found lower CoQ10 levels in people who have cancer, compared to those who do not.

Early research suggests that CoQ10 in combination with other antioxidants may increase survival in end-stage cancer. However, more information is needed on CoQ10 alone.

Low levels of CoQ10 may be linked to risk of breast cancer. There is promising evidence to support the use of CoQ10 in the treatment of breast cancer, possibly in combination with conventional therapy.

Early study reports that CoQ10 in combination with vitamin E, vitamin C, and conventional therapy may reduce the dosage of asthma medication required.

CoQ10 has been studied for use as an antioxidant to protect cells from damage. CoQ10 has been used in combination with other antioxidants. Early study suggests that it may have antioxidant benefits in people with heart disease. **RMH Note: Please remember that CoQ10 can also serve as a prooxidant, just as with many other so-called antioxidants.**

There is some evidence that idebenone, a man-made compound similar to CoQ10, may benefit people with Alzheimer's disease. However, the effect of CoQ10 itself is unclear.

Early study suggests that a combination of CoQ10 and other anti-oxidants and minerals may improve skin roughness and fine wrinkles. Further research is needed to understand CoQ10's role in skin aging.

Age-related macular degeneration (AMD) is an eye condition that causes vision loss in older adults. Early research suggests that a combination of acetyl-L-carnitine, omega-3, and CoQ10 may improve visual function in early AMD. More research is needed on the effects of CoQ10 alone.

There is good evidence to support the use of CoQ10 in the treatment of high blood pressure. However, more studies evaluating a higher dose for a longer treatment period are needed.

Negative aspects of CoQ10

Also, **the Mayo Clinic website lists as "unclear" the use of CoQ10 with antiaging, asthma, breast cancer, eye health, cataracts, chemotherapy side effects, chest pain, chronic fatigue syndrome, cocaine dependence, coronary heart disease, cystic fibrosis, dry mouth, exercise performance, fibromyalgia, gum disease, hearing loss, heart attack, chronic myocardial disease, heart disease prevention, heart muscle injury, high cholesterol, HIV/AIDS, hypertriglyceridemia, immune enhancement, infant development/neonatal care, kidney failure, male infertility, migraine, mitochondrial diseases, mitral valve prolapse, movement disorders, muscle weakness, muscular dystrophies, myelodysplastic syndrome, nerve pain, Parkinson's disease, Peyronie's disease, pre-eclampsia, prostate cancer, psoriasis, recovery from surgery, ringing in the ears and weight loss.**

Early evidence supports the use of CoQ10 in the treatment of heart-related complications in people with diabetes. However, overall study results suggest that CoQ10 may lack effect on blood sugar control.

Limited research reports that CoQ10 may lack benefit in people who have hepatitis C.

There is negative evidence to support the use of CoQ10 or idebenone (a man-made compound similar to CoQ10) for the treatment of Huntington's disease.

A combination product containing CoQ10 lacked benefit in men with prostate cancer.

Results are conflicting in support of CoQ10 for the treatment of kidney failure.

Early research suggests that evidence is lacking to support of the use of CoQ10 for treating HIV/AIDS.

Evidence is conflicting in support of the cholesterol-lowering effects of CoQ10.

There is unclear evidence to support the use of CoQ10 for side effects of chemotherapy on the heart.

Early study suggests that CoQ10 may benefit eye health. CoQ10 has been used in combination with vitamin A to improve nerve regeneration in the eye. However, the effect of CoQ10 alone is unclear.

Coenzyme Q10 for heart failure

Abstract

BACKGROUND:

Coenzyme Q10, or ubiquinone, is a non-prescription nutritional supplement. It is a fat-soluble molecule that acts as an electron carrier in mitochondria and as a coenzyme for mitochondrial enzymes. Coenzyme Q10 deficiency may be associated with a multitude of diseases including heart failure. The severity of heart failure correlates with the severity of coenzyme Q10 deficiency. Emerging data suggest that the harmful effects of reactive oxygen species are increased in patients with heart failure and coenzyme Q10 may help to reduce these toxic effects because of its antioxidant activity. **RMH Note: Actually, CoQ10 is a good prooxidant.** Coenzyme Q10 may also have a role in stabilizing myocardial calcium-dependent ion channels and preventing the consumption of metabolites essential for adenosine-5'-triphosphate (ATP) synthesis. Coenzyme Q10, although not a primary recommended treatment, could be beneficial to patients with heart failure. **Several randomized controlled trials have compared coenzyme Q10 to other therapeutic modalities, but no systematic review of existing randomized trials has been conducted.** (Madmani et al, 2014)

OBJECTIVES:

To review the safety and efficacy of coenzyme Q10 in heart failure.

SEARCH METHODS:

We searched the Cochrane Central Register of Controlled Trials (CENTRAL) (2012, Issue 12); MEDLINE OVID (1950 to January Week 3 2013) and EMBASE OVID (1980 to 2013 Week 03) on 24 January 2013; Web of Science with Conference Proceedings (1970 to January 2013) and CINAHL Plus (1981 to January 2013) on 25 January 2013; and AMED (Allied and Complementary Medicine) (1985 to January 2013) on 28 January 2013. We applied no language restrictions.

SELECTION CRITERIA:

We included randomized controlled trials of either parallel or cross-over design that assessed the beneficial and harmful effects of coenzyme Q10 in patients with heart failure. When cross-over studies were identified, we considered data only from the first phase.

DATA COLLECTION AND ANALYSIS:

Two authors independently extracted data from the included studies onto a pre-designed data extraction form. We then entered the data into Review Manager 5.2 for analysis. We assessed study risk of bias using the Cochrane 'Risk of bias' tool. For dichotomous data, we calculated the risk ratio and for continuous data the mean difference (MD). Where appropriate data were available, we performed meta-analysis. For this review we prioritised data from pooled analyses only. Where meta-analysis was not possible, we wrote a narrative synthesis. We provided a QUOROM flow chart to show the flow of papers.

MAIN RESULTS:

We included seven studies with 914 participants comparing coenzyme Q10 versus placebo. There were no data on clinical events from published randomized trials. The included studies had small sample sizes. Meta-analysis was only possible for a few physiological measures and there was substantial heterogeneity. Only one study reported on total mortality, major cardiovascular events and hospitalization. Five trials reported on the New York Heart Association (NYHA) classification of clinical status, but it was impossible to pool data due to heterogeneity.

None of the included trials considered quality of life, exercise variables, adverse events or cost-effectiveness as outcome measures. **Pooled analysis suggests that the use of coenzyme Q10 has no clear effect on left ventricular ejection fraction or exercise capacity**. Pooled data did indicate that supplementation increased blood levels of coenzyme Q10. However, there are only a small number of small studies with a risk of bias, so these results should be interpreted with caution.

AUTHORS' CONCLUSIONS:

No conclusions can be drawn on the benefits or harms of coenzyme Q10 in heart failure at this time (2014), as trials published to date lack information on clinically relevant endpoints. Furthermore, the existing data are derived from small, heterogeneous trials that concentrate on physiological measures: **their results are inconclusive**. Until further evidence emerges to support the use of coenzyme Q10 in heart failure, there might be a need to re-evaluate whether further trials testing coenzyme Q10 in heart failure are desirable. (Madmani et al, 2014)

CoQ10 for prevention of cardiovascular disease

Abstract

BACKGROUND:

Cardiovascular disease (CVD) remains the number one cause of death and disability worldwide and public health interventions focus on modifiable risk factors, such as diet. Coenzyme Q10 (CoQ10) is an antioxidant that is naturally synthesized by the body and can also be taken as a dietary supplement. Studies have shown that a CoQ10 deficiency is associated with cardiovascular disease.

OBJECTIVES:

To determine the effects of coenzyme Q10 supplementation as a single ingredient for the primary prevention of CVD.

SEARCH METHODS:

We searched the Cochrane Central Register of Controlled Trials (CENTRAL 2013, Issue 11); MEDLINE (Ovid, 1946 to November week

3 2013); EMBASE (Ovid, 1947 to 27 November 2013) and other relevant resources on 2 December 2013. We applied no language restrictions.

SELECTION CRITERIA:

Randomized controlled trials (RCTs) lasting at least three months involving healthy adults or those at high risk of CVD but without a diagnosis of CVD. Trials investigated the supplementation of CoQ10 alone as a single supplement. The comparison group was no intervention or placebo. The outcomes of interest were CVD clinical events and major CVD risk factors, adverse effects and costs. We excluded any trials involving multifactorial lifestyle interventions to avoid confounding.

DATA COLLECTION AND ANALYSIS:

Two authors independently selected trials for inclusion, abstracted data and assessed the risk of bias. We contacted authors for additional information where necessary.

MAIN RESULTS

We identified six RCTs with a total of 218 participants randomized, one trial awaiting classification and five ongoing trials. All trials were conducted in participants at high risk of CVD, two trials examined CoQ10 supplementation alone and four examined CoQ10 supplementation in patients on statin therapy; we analyzed these separately. **All six trials were small-scale**, recruiting between 20 and 52 participants; one trial was at high risk of bias for incomplete outcome data and one for selective reporting; **all studies were unclear in the method of allocation and therefore for selection bias**. The dose of CoQ10 varied between 100 mg/day and 200 mg/day and the duration of the interventions was similar at around three months. No studies reported mortality or non-fatal cardiovascular events. None of the included studies provided data on adverse events. Two trials examined the effect of CoQ10 on blood pressure. For systolic blood pressure we did not perform a meta-analysis due to significant heterogeneity. **In one trial CoQ10 supplementation had no effect on systolic blood pressure**.

In the other trial there was a statistically significant reduction in systolic blood pressure.

For diastolic blood pressure we performed a random-effects meta-analysis, which showed no evidence of effect of CoQ10 supplementation when these two small trials were pooled.

One trial (51 patients randomized) looked at the effect of CoQ10 on lipid levels. **The trial showed no evidence of effect of CoQ10 supplementation on total cholesterol, high-density lipoprotein (HDL)-cholesterol or triglycerides.**

Of the four trials that investigated CoQ10 supplementation in patients on statin therapy, **three of them showed that simultaneous administration of CoQ10 did not significantly influence lipid levels or systolic blood pressure levels** between the two groups.

The fourth trial showed a significant increase in the change in total and low-density lipoprotein (LDL)-cholesterol at three months across the four arms of the trial (α-tocopherol, CoQ10, CoQ10 + α-tocopherol and placebo), however the way in which the data were presented meant that we were unable to determine if there was any significant difference between the CoQ10 only and placebo arms.

In contrast, **there was no significant difference in the change in HDL-cholesterol and triglycerides after three months between the four arms of the trial**.

AUTHORS' CONCLUSIONS:

There are very few studies to date examining CoQ10 for the primary prevention of CVD. The results from the ongoing studies will add to the evidence base. Due to the small number of underpowered trials contributing to the analyses, **the results presented should be treated with caution** and further high quality trials with longer-term follow-up are needed to determine the effects on cardiovascular events. (Flowers et al, 2014)

CoQ10 in pulmonary arterial hypertension

Abstract

Mitochondrial dysfunction is a fundamental abnormality in the vascular endothelium and smooth muscle of patients with pulmonary arterial hypertension (PAH). Because coenzyme Q (CoQ) is essential for mitochondrial function and efficient oxygen utilization as the electron carrier in the inner mitochondrial membrane, we hypothesized that CoQ would improve mitochondrial function and benefit PAH patients.

To test this, oxidized and reduced levels of CoQ, cardiac function by echocardiogram, mitochondrial functions of heme synthesis and cellular metabolism were evaluated in PAH patients (N=8) in comparison to healthy controls (N=7), at baseline and after 12 weeks oral CoQ supplementation. *CoQ levels were similar among pulmonary arterial hypertension (PAH) and control individuals, and increased in all subjects with CoQ supplementation.*

PAH patients had higher CoQ levels than controls with supplementation, and a tendency to a higher reduced-to-oxidized CoQ ratio. **Cardiac parameters improved with CoQ supplementation**, although **6-minute walk distances and BNP levels did not significantly change**. Consistent with improved mitochondrial synthetic function, hemoglobin increased and red cell distribution width (RDW) decreased in PAH patients with CoQ, while hemoglobin declined slightly and RDW did not change in healthy controls. In contrast, **metabolic and redox parameters, including lactate, pyruvate and reduced or oxidized gluthathione, did not change in PAH patients with CoQ**.

In summary, **CoQ improved hemoglobin and red cell maturation in PAH**, but longer studies and/or higher doses with a randomized placebo-controlled controlled design are necessary to evaluate the clinical benefit of this simple nutritional supplement. (Sharp et al, 2014)

CoQ10 has no significant effect on arterial endothelial function

CoQ10 improves LDL resistance to ex vivo oxidation but does not enhance endothelial function in hypercholesterolemic young adults.

Abstract

Oxidative modification of low-density lipoprotein (LDL) may cause arterial endothelial dysfunction in hyperlipidemic subjects. **Antioxidants can protect LDL from oxidation and therefore improve endothelial function**. Dietary supplementation with coenzyme Q (CoQ(10)) raises its level within LDL, which may subsequently become more resistant to oxidation. Therefore, the aim of this study was to assess whether oral supplementation of CoQ(10) (50 mg three times

Prof Randolph M Howes MD,PhD

daily) is effective in reducing ex vivo LDL oxidizability and in improving vascular endothelial function. Twelve nonsmoking healthy adults with hypercholesterolemia (age 34+/-10 years, nine women and three men, total cholesterol 7.4+/-1.1 mmol/l) and endothelial dysfunction (below population mean) at baseline were randomized to receive CoQ(10) or matching placebo in a double-blind crossover study (active/placebo phase 4 weeks, washout 4 weeks). Flow-mediated (FMD, endothelium-dependent) and nitrate-mediated (NMD, smooth muscle-dependent) arterial dilatation were measured by high-resolution ultrasound. **CoQ(10) treatment increased plasma CoQ(10) levels from 1.1 +/-0.5 to 5.0+/-2.8 micromol/l but had no significant effect on Flow-mediated (FMD, endothelium-dependent) and nitrate-mediated (NMD, smooth muscle-dependent) arterial dilatation or serum LDL-cholesterol levels.**

Four subjects were selected randomly for detailed analysis of LDL oxidizability using aqueous peroxyl radicals as the oxidant. In this subgroup, CoQ(10) supplementation significantly increased the time for CoQ(10) H(2) depletion upon oxidant exposure of LDL by 41+/-19 min and decreased the extent of lipid hydroperoxide accumulation after 2 hours by 50+/-37 micromol/l.

We conclude that dietary supplementation with CoQ(10) decreases ex-vivo LDL oxidizability but has no significant effect on arterial endothelial function in patients with moderate hypercholesterolemia. (Raitakari et al, 2000)

CoQ10 and vascular endothelial function: Meta-analysis of RCTs

Abstract

OBJECTIVE:

The purpose of this study was to quantify the effect of coenzyme Q10 on arterial endothelial function in patients with and without established cardiovascular disease.

BACKGROUND:

Endothelial dysfunction has been implicated in the pathogenesis of atherosclerosis.

METHODS AND RESULTS:

The search included MEDLINE, Cochrane Library, Scopus, and EMBASE to identify studies up to 1 July 2011. Eligible studies were randomized controlled trials on the effects of coenzyme Q10 compared with placebo on endothelial function. Two reviewers extracted data on study characteristics, methods, and outcomes. Five eligible trials enrolled a total of 194 patients. Meta-analysis using random-effects model showed treatment with **coenzyme Q10 significantly improvement in endothelial function assessed peripherally by flow-mediated dilatation.** However, **the endothelial function assessed peripherally by nitrate-mediated arterial dilatation was not significantly improved with CoQ10 by using fix-effects model.**

CONCLUSION:

Coenzyme Q10 supplementation is associated with significant improvement in endothelial function. The current study supports a role for CoQ10 supplementation in patients with endothelial dysfunction. (Gao et al, 2011)

Does CoQ10 protect endothelial cells from beta-amyloid uptake?

Coenzyme Q10 protects human endothelial cells from β-amyloid uptake and oxidative stress-induced injury.

Abstract

Neuropathological symptoms of Alzheimer's disease appear in advanced stages, once neuronal damage arises. Nevertheless, recent studies demonstrate that in early asymptomatic stages, ß-amyloid peptide damages the cerebral microvasculature through mechanisms that involve an increase in reactive oxygen species and calcium, which induces necrosis and apoptosis of endothelial cells, leading to cerebrovascular dysfunction. The goal of our work is to study the potential preventive effect of the lipophilic antioxidant coenzyme Q (CoQ) against ß-amyloid-induced damage on human endothelial cells. We analyzed the protective effect of CoQ against Aß-induced injury in human umbilical vein endothelial cells (HUVECs) using fluorescence and confocal microscopy, biochemical techniques and RMN-based metabolomics. Our results show that **CoQ pretreatment of HUVECs delayed Aβ incorporation into the plasma membrane and mitochondria.**

Moreover, **CoQ reduced the influx of extracellular Ca(2+), and Ca(2+) release from mitochondria due to opening the mito-chondrial transition pore after β-amyloid administration, in addition to decreasing O2(.-) and H2O2 levels.**

Pretreatment with **CoQ also prevented ß-amyloid-induced HUVECs necrosis and apoptosis, restored their ability to pro-liferate, migrate and form tube-like structures in vitro, which is mirrored by a restoration of the cell metabolic profile to control levels.**

CoQ protected endothelial cells from Aβ-induced injury at physiological concentrations in human plasma after oral CoQ supplementation and thus could be a promising molecule to protect endothelial cells against amyloid angiopathy. However, this was a totally in vitro study. (Duran-Prado et al, 2014)

CoQ10 effects in alloxan type-1 diabetic rats

Antiatherogenic, hepatoprotective, and hypolipidemic effects of coenzyme Q10 in alloxan-induced type I diabetic rats.

Abstract

BACKGROUND:

Diabetes mellitus, one of the leading metabolic syndromes, accounts for highest morbidity and mortality worldwide. In this study, we examined possible protective effect of coenzyme Q10 on lipid profile, atherogenic index, and liver enzyme markers in alloxan-induced type I diabetic rats.

METHODS:

A total of **30 male rats** were randomly divided into three groups; group 1 as control, group 2 diabetic untreatment, and group 3 treat-ments with coenzyme Q10 by 15 mg/kg i.p. daily, respectively. Diabetes was induced in the second and third groups by alloxan injection sub-cutaneously. After 8 weeks, the levels of fasting blood glucose (FBG), triglyceride (TG), total cholesterol (TC), low density lipoprotein (LDL), very low-density lipoprotein (VLDL), high density lipoprotein (HDL), atherogenic index, atherogenic coefficient, cardiac risk ratio, and the activities of alanine aminotransferase (ALT), aspartate aminotransferase (AST), and alkaline phosphatase (ALP) of all groups were analyzed. Data were analyzed using non-parametric Mann-Whitney test (using SPSS) and $P < 0.05$ was considered as significant.

RESULTS:

Coenzyme Q10 inhibited significantly the activities of ALT (11.17%), AST (19.35%) and ALP (36.67%) and decreased FBG (21.19%), TG (37.24%), TC (17.15%), LDL (30.44%), VLDL (37.24%), atherogenic index (44.24%), atherogenic coefficient (49.69%), and cardiac risk ratio (37.97%), HDL level was significantly (33.38%) increased when treated with coenzyme Q10.

CONCLUSION:

The findings of this study suggest that **coenzyme Q10 exert beneficial effects on the lipid profile, atherogenic index, and liver enzymes activity in alloxan-induced type 1 diabetic rats.** (Ahmadvand, Ghaseme-Dehnoo, 2014)

----

http://medshadow.org/features/side-effects-5-drugs-se-niorscommonly-take/coq-10-poses-drug-interaction-risk/

CoQ-10 Poses Drug Interaction Risk —Laura Broadwell

Coenzyme Q-10 (CoQ-10) is a natural antioxidant made by our bodies and found in foods such as fatty fish (salmon and tuna), meats and chicken, peanuts, and canola and soybean oils. Our bodies need CoQ-10 to protect cells, reduce the risk of developing chronic diseases, and convert food into energy.

But as we age, our levels of CoQ-10 start to diminish. Certain drugs such as statins (used to lower cholesterol) and beta-blockers (for high blood pressure) can also decrease our CoQ-10 levels, as can health conditions such as heart disease, high blood pressure, diabetes, and cancer. (CoQ-10 levels can be checked by a blood test; but some symptoms include muscle weakness and pain particularly for those taking statins.)

To compensate for these deficiencies—and to offset a host of other problems, including migraines, chronic fatigue, male infertility, and gum disease — millions of people worldwide take CoQ-10 supplements. **The U.S. and European market is expected to top $133 million by 2015, according to a report by Global Industry Analysts**.

But seniors who consume CoQ-10 supplements need to exercise caution: These nutraceuticals can cause problems if combined with other drugs. For example, since **CoQ-10 has a relaxing effect on blood vessels, it can lower blood pressure levels.** *If taken with a high blood pressure medication, CoQ-10 can cause blood pressure to drop too low*.

Speaking to The New York Times, Roxanne Sukol, MD, a preventive medicine specialist at the Cleveland Clinic's Wellness Institute, says, "It takes about eight weeks for this effect to kick in, and those who are already on blood pressure medications and choose to take CoQ-10 should do so under the guidance of a doctor."

CoQ-10 can also reduce the effectiveness of blood thinners such as heparin, warfarin, or even aspirin. While these drugs are used to slow blood clotting, CoQ-10 can have the opposite effect, putting a senior at risk for dangerous blood clots. If a senior is taking a CoQ-10 supplement, it's important that he or she have their blood checked regularly as the dose of a blood thinner might need to be changed.

Seniors should always tell their physician about their supplement use, particularly if they are taking CoQ-10 in addition to a statin, blood thinner, or beta-blocker.

Coenzyme Q10 - By Kevin Boyd

Coenzyme Q10 (CoQ10, also called ubiquinone) is a vitamin-like substance that's present in foods and is also produced by your cells to help convert food into energy. The Japanese were the first to start taking it in supplement form, and it's still commonly used in Japan to treat heart-failure patients. **During the 1980s, CoQ10 gained popularity in this country as an energy-booster; it's now touted as an anti-aging supplement, as well as a treatment for gum disease, heart disease, and even brain disorders**.

What is it good for?

Several human studies found that CoQ10 improved the quality of life of people with congestive heart failure (CHF) above the benefit of the prescription heart medicine they took. However, **research is not consistent and the American Heart Association does not recommend CoQ10 for people with congestive heart failure**.

Limited human research suggests that CoQ10 may help some people with migraines, high blood pressure (hypertension) and muscular dystrophy. Other human research suggests it may help boost the immune systems of people with HIV infection and decrease the risk of heart problems in people who have had heart attacks. **Human studies have shot down the theory that extra CoQ10 can boost your energy or endurance or help treat gum disease.** (Watts, 1995)

Animal studies have suggested that CoQ10 might combat brain deterioration in Alzheimer's patients, but results in humans are disappointing so far. A small government study reported in the Archives of Neurology suggests that CoQ10 may slow the rate of functional decline in people with early-stage Parkinson's disease. However, researchers caution that more research is needed to bear this out.

A number of prescription medicines (beta-blockers, statins and some oral anti-diabetes drugs) can lower CoQ10 levels in the body. Some people think that it is a good idea to take CoQ10 supplements to boost the levels, **but there are no human studies to show if this is necessary or even a good idea.**

How does it work?

Coenzyme Q10 grabs the electrons that are generated as you digest food and shuttles them around inside the cells, a process that helps to produce energy. Researchers theorize that heart-disease patients may not make enough CoQ10 and that supplements can help keep their stressed hearts pumping. CoQ10 may function as an antioxidant, a substance which neutralizes harmful free radicals by supplying their missing electrons, so they don't go stealing electrons from cells and thus causing the kind of cell damage that leads to cancer and other diseases.

How safe is it?

CoQ10 rarely causes side effects. *Occasionally, it causes stomach upset or diarrhea, especially when more than 100 milligrams* *is taken in a single dose*. But be aware that the government doesn't regulate supplements, so there's no guarantee of their safety or effectiveness. Even though CoQ10 has been studied for 45 years, no research has looked at its long-term effects. *CoQ10 can reduce the effect of the blood thinner Coumadin (Warfarin)*. People on Warfarin therapy should talk with their doctor before taking CoQ10. (Spigset, 1994)

How is it taken?

You can buy coenzyme Q10 at almost any health-food store, at many supermarkets, and over the Internet. It's usually sold in the form of tablets or capsules, or in combination with vitamins or other substances (such as lecithin) as a healthy-heart supplement. Advocates suggest that you take 100 to 150 mg of CoQ10 daily to combat heart disease. But check with your doctor before taking any new supplement. Be aware that the government doesn't regulate supplements as it does drugs. There's no required testing for safety and effectiveness, for example. Quality and potency can vary from product to product, so ask a pharmacist or naturopath to recommend a reputable brand.

Coenzyme Q10 for heart failure: The hype and the science

Posted by Scott Gavura on June 20, 2013

Could a product sold as a dietary supplement really be delivering the benefits that advocates have claimed for decades? That's what you might be wondering about coenzyme Q10, following recent stories like:

- **The energy-boosting supplement that could HALVE the number of deaths from heart failure** screamed *The Daily Mail*.

- **It's Official: Coenzyme Q10 Improves Heart Failure Survival** from the "orthomolecular" advocates AOR.

- **Could Antioxidant Supplement Cut Heart Failure Risk?** asked eMaxHealth.

- **First Drug to Significantly Improve Heart Failure Mortality in Over a Decade** from Live Science.

- **Could supplements be the key to boosting survival from heart failure?** asked WebMD.

What's caused all the excitement about CoQ10 is **the Q-SYMBIO trial**, more properly called **"The effect of coenzyme Q10 on morbidity and mortality in chronic heart failure"**, presented at the European Society of Cardiology conference.

Coenzyme Q10 (CoQ10) has a long and mixed history filled with both promise and disappointment. Also known as vitamin Q10, ubiquinone, or ubidecarenone, **CoQ10 isn't actually vitamin, as the body produces its own supply**.

CoQ10 is found in most cells of the body, with high concentrations in the heart, liver, kidney, and pancreas. Its function seems to include antioxidant effects as well as acting as a cofactor in multiple metabolic pathways. **Supplementation can push blood levels much higher than anything the body can produce on its own**.

While trials with supplements have been small and somewhat equivocal, **CoQ10 seems to effectively treat rare cases of coenzyme Q-10 deficiency, as well as conditions resulting in mitochondrial deficiencies.** At least one formulation of CoQ10 has been FDA-approved as an orphan drug for the treatment of these rare disorders.

The majority of the CoQ10 research has focused on cardiovascular disease such as congestive heart failure and angina, but there is also some limited study of its use in diabetes, hypertension, chronic fatigue, and a long list of other conditions.

Finally there's the question of whether it's useful for preventing "statin"-drug-induced muscle pain, where the bottom line seems to be "**maybe**".

In general, most of the studies have been poorly designed and had small sample sizes, giving lots of results which are promising but little that is unambiguously positive.

This hasn't stopped advocates, particularly supplement vendors, from recommending it as a panacea for just about anything, and even adding it to products like cosmetics.

Given what appears to be a reasonably good safety profile, CoQ10 is a supplement advocate's dream: a "natural" product that seems safe and may actually work.

But is CoQ10 actually a supplement at all? The line between supplements and therapeutic drugs isn't an easy one to define.

Vitamins can be treated like drugs (e.g., niacin) and some drugs are rebranded as supplements if they can't pass the evidence standards to be approved drug products. **Natural substances can be marketed as both supplements and drugs** (e.g., magnesium) or as drugs alone (e.g., epinephrine). There is not always a clear line, and the variations between countries can be striking.

It generally seems to be based more on evaluations of safety than that of efficacy. This may in part explain the varying use of CoQ10 around the world. It's probably most widely used in Japan, which coincidentally is also the world's biggest supplier.

There it's apparently used as a routine treatment for congestive heart failure, where it was approved for this purpose almost 40 years ago. It's also used Europe and Russia, though **the U.S. and Japanese markets make up 85% of the world's consumption**.

Supplement or drug, what matters is whether it works when it's evaluated using objective standards. So describing a supplement like CoQ10 as an "alternative" or "complementary" treatment for heart failure is using misleading terminology.

As has been said before, there is no such thing as alternative medicine: There is medicine, which are treatments shown to work, and treatments which are unproven to work, or proven not to work. Medicine does not fail to work in a conventional sense and yet work in some "alternative" sense.

The study

It has not been established that CoQ10 helps in heart failure, but smaller studies have shown improvements in exercise tolerance and other measures, though not consistently.

Observed benefits may be due to the prevention of oxidative damage (antioxidant) or to some other mechanism that has not yet been determined. **The evidence to date suggests that at best, CoQ10 may offer some benefit to patients already taking other drugs for heart failure but still experiencing significant disease effects.**

The current study was quite simple by design, with what appears to be a meaningful and unambiguous endpoint: major adverse cardiac event

(MACE) including hospitalization due to worsening CHF, cardiovascular death, and cardiac transplantation.

The Q-SYMBIO trial included 17 centers across 8 countries, and randomized 420 people with moderate-to-severe heart failure into two groups: One which took 100mg of CoQ10 three times daily, the other a placebo. All continued their regular medications. Patients had an average ejection fraction of 31% (that's not good) and they were, on average, 62 years of age. After two years:

- **14% on CoQ10 experienced a major adverse cardiac event, versus 25% in the placebo group (p=0.003).**

- **9% of patients on CoQ10 died, versus 17% in the placebo group (p=0.01).**

These are remarkable results for any treatment, and are particularly impressive if patients were already optimized on medical treatments (which isn't clear). And if they are validated, then CoQ10 offers a dramatic benefit to patients with heart failure. But is the effect real? Notwithstanding the fact that we don't actually have the full paper to critique, criticisms and concerns have been raised:

- The trial took over 10 years to complete, which is long for a trial with a two year endpoint, suggesting difficulty recruiting patients. The trial was first described over a decade ago.

- We don't know the medications the participants were taking, and if they would still be considered appropriate and optimal, based on today's evidence.

- The mortality rate of about 9% per year seemed low for a population this ill.

- Reporting and documentation of harms is not well described.

- The benefit seems implausibly good, and similar benefits haven't been observed in other endpoints, consistently, in other trials of CoQ10.

- What we know about how CoQ10 might work is inconsistent with what's been seen with statin trials in patients with heart failure. Statins lower CoQ10 levels, but don't worsen CHF.

- As cardiology studies go, this is a small trial. It's not clear if it was powered to detect mortality differences. The small numbers of deaths leads to imprecise estimates of risk reductions.

Coenzyme Q10 is manufactured by Pharma Nord.

Interestingly (supplement proponents and conspiracy theorists, please note) **this trial has Big Pharma's fingers all over it.** Sponsors included the International Coenzyme Q10 Association (the advocacy organization), Kaneka Corporation of Osaka (the manufacturer) and Pharma Nord (the marketer) which sells products containing coenzyme Q10.

So much for the old **trope** that pharma's trying to suppress dietary supplements, or that pharma won't study it because it's not patentable. **With the global market for the chemical estimated at $835 (?: I can not verify this figure.) billion (in 2009)**, it's not surprising that there's a lot of interest in expanding the use of this compound. The sponsorship doesn't invalidate the study, but it does make me more cautious about drawing any conclusion until the full publication is available and has been subjected to peer review.

Investigator spin

The study still hasn't been subjected to peer review, but the lead investigator is already calling for widespread use:

Professor Mortensen said: "CoQ10 is the first new medication to improve survival in chronic heart failure and it should be added to standard therapy."

and he went on, describing a mechanism of action:

"Other heart failure medications block rather than enhance cellular processes and may have side effects. Supplementation with CoQ10, which is a natural and safe substance, corrects a deficiency in the body and blocks the vicious metabolic cycle in chronic heart failure called the energy starved heart."

Natural. Safe. Mortensen has clearly drunk deeply from the CoQ10 Kool-Aid. And I can understand (in part) his enthusiasm, given the results he's reporting. But has he really found a holy grail for CHF patients? It's rare that a single trial results in a major change in medical practice. If you're a regular reader of this blog you'll know that many of us are fans of the research of John Ioannidis, particularly his work showing that **new and often exciting scientific results rarely hold up to scrutiny, and more importantly, replication**.

More simply, most published research findings are false. In particular, follow-up studies can invalidate highly-cited initial studies.

So a strong, unexpected effect in a single trial should be a red flag for skepticism. Replication is absolutely essential, and cardiologists are unlikely to endorse CoQ10 as a validated treatment until that occurs. This isn't a bias against supplements, it's good science at work. In the case of cardiology and antioxidants, there is very good reason for caution. When hype outpaces the evidence, unanticipated harms can result.

Millions took antioxidant vitamins for years thinking that they were heart healthy, when evidence eventually showed they are at best, useless, and at worst, harmful.

Risks and harms

Coenzyme Q appears to be a safe product with few harms documented. Trials consistently report no significant adverse effects. The most common manageable side effect is stomach upset, which can be reduced by dividing the dose throughout the day (as was done in this study). The other downside to the product is the cost, which can be considerable, although CoQ10 prices seem to vary dramatically between brands and there's a lack of information to help sort out the products which provide the best value-for-money.

Conclusion

Whether CoQ10 becomes an routine treatment for heart failure remains to be seen. The **Q-SYMBIO results are surprisingly good**, and for that reason, **there is good reason to be skeptical.**

The history of medicine is replete with stories of breakthrough studies that subsequently fail to be replicated.

Yet, despite knowing this, we continue to make the same mistake again and again. When something appears to be too good to be true, it almost always is. Until the Q-SYMBIO study is published and replicated, I'll remain skeptical of CoQ10's role in heart failure.

Prof Randolph M Howes MD,PhD

The resurrection of CoQ10: It's all about the money

DAVID L. KATZ, MD | MEDS | MARCH 26, 2013

A recent meta-analysis published in the *American Journal of Clinical Nutrition* suggests that coenzyme Q10 is of benefit in congestive heart failure. For those who like the idea that food and nutrients can be excellent medicine, this paper is interesting at the very least. But there is a case to be made that it is far more than that.

There is a case to be made that it is, in a word, miraculous.

For resurrection, after all, is a miracle. And according to a paper published in the *Annals of Internal Medicine* in April of 2000, coenzyme Q10 for heart failure was a dead concept. The authors reported 15 years ago that "coenzyme Q10 has been studied in randomized, blinded, and controlled studies and ... these studies have found no detectable benefit" and that "coenzyme Q10 should not be recommended for treatment of heart failure."

The final nail had been driven into the CoQ10-for-heart-failure hypothesis 13 years ago — and yet now, it's back. If that's not a miracle — then what is going on?

First, a bit of relevant orientation. The condition in question here, congestive heart failure, occurs in particular in the aftermath of one or more heart attacks (myocardial infarctions) which cause portions of the heart muscle to die for want of oxygen. Those areas stop pumping, of course, and the whole heart does its job less well.

The pumping efficiency of the heart is routinely measured using ultrasound as the "left ventricular ejection fraction" (LVEF), which, as the name suggests, is the proportion of blood the left ventricle is able to pump out of itself when it contracts. Roughly 55 to 70 percent is considered normal. High values can occur when the heart is stiff and muscle-bound, and tend to mean the heart empties well, but fills poorly. Congestive heart failure is associated with low values.

And that, in principle is where coenzyme Q10 (also known as ubiquinone, because it is all but "ubiquitous" in plants, albeit at very low concentrations) comes in. A coenzyme supports the work of one or more enzymes, and CoQ10 supports enzymes in the mitochondria, the energy generators of our cells, that transfer electrons. Perhaps you recall ATP, the body's principal form of stored energy, from high school biology. Well, CoQ10 helps us make it.

Since ATP represents stored energy muscle cells can use to contract, and inadequate contraction is the problem in congestive heart failure, it is plausible that coenzyme Q10 might help.

So, why didn't it in the April, 2000 study in the *Annals*? Well, of course it's possible that it really doesn't work. Not every good and plausible idea is right — that's why we need good science and unbiased methods. We fall all too readily in love with our own hypotheses, and only robust, objective methods can save us from that tendency.

But there's another good explanation. The study in question enrolled a total of 55 adults — of whom nine failed to finish. The study lasted a total of six months. So, in 46 adults already on what was optimal medication for congestive heart failure at the time, **CoQ10 for six months did not produce a discernible improvement in the LVEF.**

The problem with that was revealed almost exactly a year later. In May of 2001, results of the CAPRICORN trial were published in the Lancet. **CAPRICORN demonstrated that the proprietary drug carvedilol, patented and marketed as Coreg by GlaxoSmithKline, was effective in reducing mortality from congestive heart failure. It did so by enrolling nearly 2,000 patients and following them for a span of years.**

Had carvedilol been studied in 46 patients for six months, it's quite clear that nothing of consequence would have been seen. Presumably, on that basis, the final nail might have been driven into the carvedilol-for-heart-failure hypothesis. But a huge trial, costing many millions of dollars, and funded by the company that stood to profit from its results — precluded that unhappy outcome.

What would the result have been if coenzyme Q10 had been studied in 2,000 people followed for years? Nobody knows. **Since no one company can patent CoQ10, no entity is motivated to fund such a trial.** Certainly the new meta-analysis, which pools data from multiple smaller studies, suggests the results of a larger trial of CoQ10 might be very different.

Prof Randolph M Howes MD,PhD

It is well established that much, even most, of what constitutes conventional medicine is just tradition and not truly evidence-based by today's standards. My own work in evidence mapping, a technique colleagues and I invented that was subsequently adopted by the World Health Organization, reveals that the evidence base underlying practices in CAM is quite diverse. The simple summary of it all is that there is both baby and bathwater in CAM and conventional medicine alike, and it requires open-mindedness and unbiased methods to distinguish between them.

It also requires money, which brings us full circle.

Reports of nails in CAM's coffin tend to be premature — because the many unpatentable modalities in the realm of CAM do not inspire huge and costly trials. We need such trials to know for sure what does and doesn't work. I believe at this point that CoQ10 is beneficial in heart failure — but don't know for sure.

The story of CoQ10's resurrection for heart failure across a span of more than a decade is in fact, not a tale of miracles. **It's all about money**.

David L. Katz is the founding director of Yale University's Prevention Research Center.

CoQ10 Strikes Out in Phase 3 for Parkinson's

31 Mar 2014

http://www.alzforum.org/news/research-news/coenzyme-q10-strikes-out-phase-3-parkinsons. Accessed 5-29-14.

Coenzyme Q10 treatment does not slow the progression of Parkinson's disease (PD). This was the disappointing conclusion of a Phase 3 clinical trial designed to test the disease-modifying potential of the drug.

CoQ10 is an antioxidant that supports mitochondrial function. The results, **published March 24, 2014 in JAMA Neurology**, come on the heels of a promising Phase 2 study, but **also amid negative outcomes from other small trials of this compound**. The large, multicenter trial, called **"QE3," likely puts an end to hopes of**

using coenzyme Q10 to treat sporadic PD, said Flint Beal of Weill Cornell Medical College in New York, the trial's lead investigator. "We are quite **disappointed**, but we can't argue with the data," he told Alzforum.

No Brakes on Parkinson's Progression: Treatment with coenzyme Q10 failed to curb PD in a phase 3 clinical trial. Parkinson's progression scores climbed at an equal pace in treatment groups (blue) and placebo group (orange) over the 16-month trial period. [Copyright © 2014 American Medical Association. All rights reserved.]

Also called ubiquinone, coenzyme Q10 is a component of the electron transport chain that drives the generation of ATP in mitochondria.

CoQ10 accepts electrons from Complex I, a 46-subunit machine that pumps protons across the inner mitochondrial membrane, and hands the electrons off to the next member of the respiratory chain.

Thus reduced, CoQ10 acts as a powerful antioxidant and has been shown to counteract oxidative damage, a form of injury associated with neurodegenerative disease.

Researchers hoped that the coenzyme would stave off damage to dopaminergic neurons in people with PD. Animal studies suggested the approach held promise. (Spindler et al, 2009)

QE3's smaller predecessor trial, **QE2, gave researchers reason for optimism**, as well. In that North American multicenter Phase 2 trial, 80 people newly diagnosed with Parkinson's disease received one of three daily doses (300, 600, or 1200 mg) of CoQ10 or a placebo. All groups also took Vitamin E, owing to previous reports that the lipophilic vitamin may enhance CoQ10 uptake and have synergistic antioxidant effects. The participants were monitored for signs of disease progression for 16 months, or until their PD had progressed to a point where they had to start dopaminergic therapy. In this small trial, **treatment appeared to correlate with slowed disease progression in a dose-dependent manner**, a finding that stimulated researchers to move forward with the larger QE3 trial. (Shults et al, 2002)

The QE3 trial spanned 67 treatment centers that together enrolled 600 patients. The larger trial followed the same protocol as QE2 but upped the dose; the participants were given either 1200 mg or 2400 mg. At both these higher doses, CoQ10 was generally well tolerated and triggered minimal adverse events, the scientists report. However, **disease symptoms progressed just as quickly in both CoQ10 groups as in the placebo group. The investigators concluded that CoQ10 showed no evidence of benefit in early Parkinson's Disease patients.**

"I'm really puzzled by it—the QE2 trial looked so good," said David Simon, the lead trial investigator at Beth Israel Deaconess Medical Center in Boston. "But there's a reason why we do not move directly from small Phase 2 studies into clinical practice. They don't always replicate."

Despite the QE2 trial results, two other studies completed after the initiation of the QE3 trial had already begun to temper expectations.

In 2007, the National Institute of Neurological Disorders and Stroke Neuroprotection Exploratory Trials (NET-PD) consortium tested 2400 mg CoQ10 in PD patients. (NET-PD, 2007)

A primary analysis of the results, which relied on historical controls, deemed CoQ10 worthy of moving into a larger trial. **However, a secondary analysis using controls that more closely resembled the treatment group found that continuing with the drug would be futile.**

By this point, the QE3 trial had already been funded, Simon said. Another recent trial tested MitoQ, a chemically modified version of CoQ10 designed to efficiently cross cellular membranes and target the mitochondria. **This study was negative, as well (see Snow et al., 2010).** (Snow et al, 2010)

In spite of the rash of failures with CoQ10, Simon still believes that targeting the mitochondria is a solid approach to treating PD. "The data implicating mitochondrial dysfunction as a cause of PD is overwhelming," he said. Simon added that the variety of causes that underlie sporadic PD, and the lack of biomarkers available to stratify them, may make it difficult to identify the patients most likely to benefit from such treatments.

For example, a recent study found that mutations in PINK1, which are known to cause PD, prevented the ability of Complex I to pass electrons off to CoQ10 in the respiratory chain (see Mar 2014 news story). The transfer is necessary to drive the proton gradient that generates ATP. "If you were to give CoQ10 to patients with PINK1 mutations, it would not bind or receive electrons from Complex I, so it would not help," said that study's leader, Bart De Strooper of the University of Leuven in Belgium. However, De Strooper added that patients with different mitochondrial defects theoretically could have benefited from the treatment. "I don't think the trial is definitive. It only shows that the treatment won't work in the broad population of sporadic PD patients," he said.

The QE3 study investigators were unable to determine whether CoQ10 reached its target in the brain. They also do not know if whatever fraction of CoQ10 that did get into the brain improved mitochondrial function there. An analysis of blood mitochondrial activity in the QE2 trial indicated that CoQ10 enhanced respiratory chain function, however, that analysis was not done in the QE3 trial. "**We think of CoQ10 as a mitochondrial drug, but what it really does and where it actually goes is not clear**," said Russell Swerdlow of the University of Kansas Medical Center, Kansas City. If it does make it to the brain and into the mitochondria, "does it prevent oxidative damage, enhance the respiratory chain, or perhaps do neither of those things?" Swerdlow asked.

In Alzheimer's disease, most clinical trials in the past decade were negative, and many of those trials did not rigorously quantify drug exposure and target engagement.

Swerdlow added, however, that the QE3 trial was a reasonable attempt to treat mitochondrial dysfunction, which he sees as a major cause of sporadic PD. Swerdlow has his sights set on other ways to improve mitochondrial function, such as treatment with oxaloacetate, a bioenergetic intermediate that changes the redox balance of the mitochondria and promotes respiration.

CoQ10 is commercially available as a food supplement. Flint agrees that though QE3 has dashed hopes of treating PD with CoQ10, enhancing mitochondrial function still holds promise. "There are a lot of creative approaches being developed," he said. For example, **Flint and colleagues have treated animal models with mitochondrial-targeted peptides that protect dopaminergic neurons from death**. (Yang et al, 2009)

On this point, Anthony Schapira and Sandip Patel of University College London pose a rhetorical question in an accompanying editorial: "Is this the end of the road for targeting mitochondria for neuroprotection in PD? Our answer to this would be an unequivocal 'no.'"—Jessica Shugart

CoQ10 did not result in improved self-reported fatigue or QOL

Abstract

BACKGROUND:

Coenzyme Q10 (CoQ10) is a common antioxidant supplement with known cardioprotective effects and potential anticancer benefits.

OBJECTIVES:

We performed a randomized, double-blind, placebo-controlled study of oral CoQ10 in female breast cancer patients with the primary objective of determining **CoQ10's effects on self-reported fatigue, depression, and quality of life (QOL)**. Methods: Eligible women with newly diagnosed breast cancer and planned adjuvant chemotherapy were randomized to oral supplements of 300 mg CoQ10 or placebo, each combined with 300 IU vitamin E, divided into 3 daily doses. **Treatment was continued for 24 weeks**. Blood tests, QOL measures, and levels of plasma CoQ10 and vitamin E were obtained at baseline and at 8, 16, and 24 weeks. Mixed-effects models were used to assess treatment differences in outcomes over time.

RESULTS:

Between September 2004 and March 2009, 236 women were enrolled. Treatment arms were well balanced with respect to age (range, 28-85 years), pathologic stage (stage 0, 91%; stage 1, 8%; stage II, 1%), ethnicity (white, 87%; black, 11%; Hispanic, 2%), and planned therapy. Baseline CoQ10 levels in the CoQ10 and placebo arms were 0.70 and 0.73 microg/mL, respectively; the 24-week CoQ10 levels were 1.83 and 0.79 microg/mL, respectively. **There were no significant differences between the CoQ10 and placebo arms at 24 weeks for scores on the Profile of Mood States-Fatigue questionnaire, the Functional Assessment of Chronic Illness Therapy-Fatigue tool, the Functional Assessment of Cancer Therapy-Breast Cancer instrument, or the Center for Epidemiologic Studies-Depression scale.**

CONCLUSIONS:

Supplementation with conventional doses of CoQ10 led to sustained increases in plasma CoQ10 levels but did not result in improved self-reported fatigue or QOL after 24 weeks of treatment. (Lesser et al, 2013) a randomized, double-blind, placebo-controlled study.

CoQ10 failed in treatment of presumed statin-induced myalgias

Abstract

Coenzyme Q10 (CoQ10) deficiency has been proposed to be causal in 3-hydroxy-3-methyl-glutaryl coenzyme A reductase inhibitor (statin)-induced myopathies. However, the clinical benefit of supplementation is unproved. The purpose of the present study was to assess the effect of CoQ10 supplementation on myalgias presumed to be caused by statins. Patients currently receiving a statin who developed new-onset myalgias in ≥ 2 extremities within 60 days of initiation or a dosage increase were eligible. Patients continued statin therapy and were **randomized** using a matched design to either CoQ10 60 mg twice daily or matching placebo. Double-blind treatment continued for 3 months, and patients completed a 10-cm visual analog scale (VAS) and the Short-Form McGill Pain Questionnaire at baseline and at each monthly visit. The primary end point was the comparison of the VAS score at 1 month. A total of 76 patients were enrolled (40 in the CoQ10 arm and 36 in the placebo arm). The mean VAS score was 6 cm at baseline in both groups. At 1 month, **no difference was seen in the mean VAS score between the 2 groups** (3.9 cm in the CoQ10 group and 4 cm in the placebo group; $p = 0.97$). However, 5 patients in the CoQ10 group and 3 in the placebo group discontinued therapy during the first month because of myalgias. The baseline median score on the Sensory Pain Rating Index subscale was 10 in the CoQ10 group and 11.5 in the placebo group. At 1 month, these scores had decreased to 6.5 and 7.5, respectively, with no statistically significant difference ($p = 0.34$).

In conclusion, **CoQ10 did not produce a greater response than placebo in the treatment of presumed statin-induced myalgias**. (Bookstaver et al, 2012)

Prof Randolph M Howes MD,PhD

CoQ10 and selenium failed to alter statin-induced myopathy (SIM)

It failed for both subjective symptoms and muscle function.

Abstract

OBJECTIVE:

The aim of the present study was to evaluate the possible effects of Q10 and selenium supplementation on statin-induced myopathy (SIM), both for subjective symptoms and muscle function.

DESIGN:

Patients (N = 43) who had experienced previous or ongoing SIM on atorvastatin therapy were recruited. Following a 6-week washout period during which no statins were administered, the patients were re-challenged with 10 mg of atorvastatin. Patients (N = 41) who experienced SIM continued the atorvastatin treatment and were in addition randomized to receive 12 weeks supplement of 400 mg Q10 and 200 µg selenium per day or a matching double placebo. SIM was assessed using 3 validated symptom questionnaires, and a muscle function test was performed at the beginning and at the end of the study.

RESULTS:

The patients receiving the active supplement experienced significant increases in their serum Q10 and selenium concentrations compared with the group receiving placebo. **No statistically significant differences in symptom questionnaire scores or muscle function tests were revealed between the groups.**

CONCLUSIONS:

Despite substantial increases in the serum Q10 and selenium levels following the oral supplementation, this study revealed no significant effects of CoQ10 and selenium on statin-induced myopathy (SIM) compared with the placebo. (Bogsrud et al, 2013)

CoQ10 decreased statin-induced myopathy (SIM)

Abstract

The objective of this study was to evaluate the possible benefits of co-enzyme Q10 and selenium supplementation administered to patients with statin-associated myopathy (SAM). Sixty eligible patients entered the pilot study. Laboratory examination (CoQ10, selenium, creatin kinase) and intensity of SAM (visual scale) were performed at baseline, after 1 month, and at the end of study at month 3. Plasma levels of CoQ10 increased from 0.81 ± 0.39 to 3.31 ± 1.72 µmol/L in the active group of patients treated by CoQ10, compared with the placebo (p = 0.001). Also, **the symptoms of SAM significantly improved in the active group: the intensity of muscle pain decreased** from 6.7 ± 1.72 to 3.2 ± 2.1; **muscle weakness decreased** from 7.0 ± 1.63 to 2.8 ± 2.34; **muscle cramps decreased** from 5.33 ± 2.06 to 1.86 ± 2.42, $p < 0.01$, $-65 \pm 28\%$); **tiredness decreased** from the initial 6.7 ± 1.34 to 1.2 ± 1.32. We did not observe any significant changes in the placebo group.

In conclusion, **supplementation of statin-treated patients with CoQ10 resulted in a decrease in the symptoms of statin-associated myopathy (SAM), both in absolute numbers and intensity.** Additional selenium supplementation was not associated with any statistically significant decrease of SAM. **However, it is not possible to draw any definite conclusions,** even though this study was carried out in double-blind fashion, because **it involved a small number of patients.** (Fedacko et al, 2013)

CoQ10 and selenium failed to prevent headaches in children

Abstract

OBJECTIVE:

To evaluate the efficacy of Coenzyme Q10 (CoQ10) supplementation in the prevention of migraine in children using a placebo-controlled, double-blinded, crossover, add-on trial.

Prof Randolph M Howes MD,PhD

BACKGROUND:

CoQ10 has been demonstrated to have efficacy in migraine prevention in adults but lacks pediatric research with more rigorous methodology. CoQ10 has been observed to be deficient in a significant number of children and adolescents presenting to tertiary headache centers. CoQ10 has the potential to modify both the inflammatory changes that occur during recurrent migraine and the alteration of mitochondrial function. A deficit of CoQ10 could thus affect the response to treatment and clinical characteristics of migraine in children and adults.

METHODS:

One-hundred-and-twenty children and adolescents with migraine headache were randomized in a crossover, double-blind, placebo-controlled, randomized, add-on study to receive a placebo or CoQ10 (100 mg) supplement for 224 days. Data for 76 patients were available at the crossover point and 50 were analyzed at the endpoint. Response to treatment, overall headache improvement, and headache disability were assessed.

RESULTS:

Both the placebo and CoQ10 groups showed reduced migraine frequency [$F_{(1, 60)}=15.68$, $p<0.001$], severity [$F_{(1, 54)}=8.09$, $p=0.006$], and duration [$F_{(1, 45)}=6.27$, $p=0.016$] over time. CoQ10 treated patients had a significantly greater improvement in frequency from subject reported baseline starting within 4 weeks of initiation. No group differences comparing the first 4 weeks of treatment with the last 4 weeks of treatment were found in migraine frequency [$F_{(1, 60)}=2.34$, $p>0.05$], severity [$F_{(1, 54)}=0.06$, $p>0.05$], or duration [$F_{(1, 45)}=0.14$, $p>0.05$].

CONCLUSIONS:

Overall, results of the study demonstrate that children and adolescents with migraine improved over time with multidisciplinary, standardized treatment regardless of supplementation with CoQ10 or placebo. There was no difference in headache outcomes between the CoQ10 and placebo groups at day 224. Due to the improvements seen in weeks 1-4, CoQ10 may lead to earlier improvement in headache severity, but given the sample size this conclusion warrants further investigation with a larger sample. (Slater et al, 2011) a randomized in a crossover, double-blind, placebo-controlled, randomized, add-on study.

200

The Radical Nature of CoQ10

CoQ10 can also exist as a radical. Based on ESR/EPR signals, **Davies and collaborators have found that the concentration of two ubisemiquinone free radicals (presumably Qi and Qo) is very high in exercised animals.** (Davies, Hochstein, 1982) (Davies KJ, Hochstein P. Ubisemiquinone radicals in liver: implications for a mitochondrial Q cycle in vivo. Biochemical and biophysical research communications. 1982 Aug 31;107(4):1292-9)

SECTION FOUR

GENERAL INFORMATION ON ANTIOXIDANTS

THE SCIENTIFIC VOYAGER

The vast immensity of the data ocean surrounds
and engulfs you.

At first, you glimpse something foggy on the far away research horizon.

You diligently pursue, in that direction, to get a better look.

A distant shape is then suggested, but needs
considerable clarification.

You move in, study it intensely - all possibilities, intensively.

An image of enlightenment begins to form.

It has a pattern and design....but is it real or just
another illusion?

More study, more study, more study and

now it congeals into focus. Your mind's eye can
see it ever so clearly.

It is a magnificent island of discovery

jutting out of a raging sea of unknowns.

Now, you must step out onto its slippery rock surface

to be scientifically satiated.

There....you feel it solidly under your feet. Eureka!

But how do you inform others of your discovery?

How do you bring them onshore with you?

Carefully, very, very carefully

for many are still blind,

still uninformed, still misinformed, still lost at sea!

Yet, for you, the tumultuous journey is at an end.

You are scientifically satisfied....

'till you launch the next inquiry.

R. M. Howes, M.D., Ph.D.

4/1/11

People the world over

want basically the same things;

adequate food, shelter, clothing,

a better life for their children, and

the instinctive urge, proclivity and propensity

to kill everyone who doesn't

look, believe and think exactly as they do.

Ahh, yes, man is the same the world over.

R.M. Howes, MD, PhD

11/29/14

An overview

First a new theory is attacked as absurd; then it is
admitted to be true, but obvious and insignificant;
finally it is seen to be so important that its adversaries
claim they themselves discovered it.
William James, *Pragmatism*, 1907

Contrary to the common mantra of many authors, oxygen free radicals perform many crucial beneficial roles in sexual function and reproduction. Also contrary to popular claims, antioxidants are not the cure-all for sexual and reproductive problems.

Before becoming a victim of antioxidant propaganda, consider the following facts I have uncovered during my decades of research:

EMODs 42 crucial roles: EMODs (electronically modified oxygen derivatives, formerly called reactive oxygen species, ROS)

EMODs
- modulate vital pathways

- control energy metabolism,

- central component of neutrophil function

- bolster survival/stress responses,

- induce apoptosis,

- manifest inflammatory response,

- regulate oxygen sensing,

- maintain redox homeostasis,

- support fertilization,

- survival kinase activation,

- ion channel regulation,

- apoptosis signaling,

- preconditioning,

- induce necrosis,

- regulate proinflammation,

- modulate the response to growth factor stimulation,

- regulation of metabolism and cytokines

- regulate vascular tone,

- induce the activity of HIF (hypoxia inducible factor)

- signal autophagy,

- generate defense against infectious agents,

- maintain vascular tone,

- control of ventilation,

- regulate erythropoietin production,

- signal transduction from membrane receptors in various physiological processes,

- act as messengers in the regulation of gene expression in development, growth, and apoptosis,

- secondary messengers in intracellular signaling cascades, which can induce the oncogenic phenotype of cancer cells, cellular senescence and apoptosis

- induce a mitogenic response,

- induce cellular senescence and apoptosis and can therefore function as anti-tumorigenic species,

- regulate development and redox homeostasis,

- participate in intracellular signaling,

- regulate "peroxide tone"

- regulate hematopoietic cells,

- regulate vascular tone via activation of guanylate cyclase,

- amplify the immune responses and apoptosis via activation of activator protein I (AP-1) and NF-κB transcription factors in human T cells,

- regulate insulin receptor kinase activity via increased activity of protein tyrosine phosphotases,

- increase expression of antioxidant enzymes and/or glutathione in response to MAPK and NF-κB activation in an effort to restore redox balance,

- a basal level of mitochondrial EMOD production appears to be essential for the attainment of a normal length lifespan,

- the level of H_2O_2 affects the expression of at least 80 different genes or proteins, including numerous components of the mitogen-activated protein kinase and nuclear factor κB signaling pathways,

- serve as metabolic intermediates in many biochemical processes including the metabolism of prostanoids, in the regulation of vasotonus, in gene regulation, e.g. activation of nuclear transcription factor kappa B (NF-kB), in the regulation of cellular growth, apoptosis and in the function of intra-as well as inter-cellular signaling and other types of signal transduction,

- modulators in most forms of cell suicide or apoptosis, the signaling cascade utilizes reactive oxygen species (EMODs) as essential intermediate messenger molecules,

- detoxifies pollutants, toxins and xenobiotics,

Here are 42 significant items involving EMODs, which demonstrate their crucial role in homeostasis and disease protection.

-- Other than that......

Oxidation reactions are crucial for all plant and animal life, and are a naturally occurring process within the cells. Such systems involve energy production, immunity, detoxification, wound healing, cellular signaling and protection against pathogens and cancer.

General Antioxidant Overview

Although I have presented over 500 studies showing non-effective or harmful effects of the antioxidant vitamins, let me give the 3 biggest pieces of evidence against their use:

1) the cumulative data of 170 studies showing harm

2) the 330 other cases showing no effect or marginal effects

3) the 5 most prevalent antioxidants in the body, when in excess, cause known disease and death, i.e., cholesterol, uric acid, bilirubin, testosterone and estrogen.

Five most obvious examples of excessive antioxidant levels: (cholesterol, uric acid, estrogen, testosterone and bilirubin are all antioxidants)

1) Hypercholesterolemia (high cholesterol)- heart disease

2) Hyperuricemia (high uric acid)- gout, gouty arthritis, heart disease

3) High estrogen levels - feeds breast cancer

4) High testosterone levels - feeds prostate cancer

5) Hyperbilirbinemia (high bilirubin levels) - causes infant jaundice and brain damage

I believe that examples of low antioxidant levels are difficult to verify, except maybe in some forms of metal poisoning.

Cancer cells concentrate protective antioxidants, lactic acid, vitamin C and glutathione.

EMOD Effects:

- modulate over 200 redox controlled genes,

- biopositive effects,

- act selectively,

- are involved in antimicrobial defense,

- involved in immunological surveillance

- are metabolic intermediates in many biochemical processes including the metabolism of prostanoids, in the regulation of vasotonus, in gene regulation, e.g. activation of nuclear transcription factor kappa B (NF-kB), in the regulation of cellular growth, apoptosis and in the function of intra- as well as inter-cellular signaling and other types of signal transduction.

- induce cellular senescence and apoptosis and can therefore function as anti-tumorigenic species (Valco et al. Int J Biochem Cell Biol. 2007).

- most forms of cell suicide or apoptosis, the signaling cascade utilizes reactive oxygen species (EMODs) as essential intermediate messenger molecules. (Slater et al, 1995) (Albright, C. D., Salganik, R. I., Craciunescu, C. N., Mar, M. H. & Zeisel, S. H. (2003).

ON A CELLULAR LEVEL:

High antioxidant levels: block the killing of bacteria, fungi, protozoans and viruses

High antioxidant levels: shield cancer cells from apoptotic death

High EMOD levels: kill bacteria, fungi, protozoans and viruses

High EMOD levels: kill cancer cells

A basal level of mitochondrial EMOD production appears to be essential for the attainment of a normal length lifespan. (Allen, Tresini, 2000)

- some removal of mitochondrial ROS can be tolerated before longevity is affected and that the increased capacity for removal of both mitochondrial $O_2^{\cdot-}$ and H_2O_2 is more harmful than for either $O_2^{\cdot-}$ or H_2O_2 alone

- the enhancement of mitochondrial antioxidative activities was associated with a decrease in lifespan

My summary of EMODs (so-called oxygen free radicals) **and antioxidants:**

Four most obvious examples of long-term low EMODs:

1) CGD (chronic granulomatous disease)- have repeated infections, granulomas (tumors) and early deaths

2) HIV/AIDS - have infections and cancer (Karposi's sarcoma)

3) Chronic steroid use - infections and cancers

4) Post chemo and radiation therapy - infections and second primary cancers

Examples of short-term low EMODs:

1) Anoxia (no oxygen): (Victims) Strangling, drowning, choking - immediate death

2) Hypoxia (low oxygen): (Pilots) CNS symptoms, dizziness, blurred vision, loss of hand-eye coordination and motor skills, hallucinations, black outs, then death

Two most obvious examples of high EMODs:

1) Exercise - best overall means of disease prevention, protection and reversal because it increases O_2 intake and EMOD production 10-15 times resting levels

2) Naked mole-rat - it is the oldest living rodent (28 yrs.), and has the highest EMOD levels, with no known cases of cancer ever reported

(Howes, 2011) (Randolph M. Howes MD, PhD. Mythology of Antioxidant Vitamins? Journal of Evidence-Based Complementary & Alternative Medicine. 2011. 16(2):149-159)

HOWES' TEN REDOX COMMANDMENTS:

1) oxygen is a electron acceptor

2) antioxidants are electron donors

3) most antioxidants have redox (prooxidant) potential

4) nearly all antioxidants can have prooxidant activity

5) most tumoricidal activity is prooxidant induced apoptosis

6) antioxidants protect cancerous cells in vitro

7) antioxidants are not antiaging agents

8) atherosclerosis is not due to EMODs

9) antioxidant overkill is dangerous, if not fatal

10) antioxidants increase overall mortality

Therapies utilizing beneficial EMODs
        Viagra, 23 millions users
        Chemotherapy, photodynamic therapy, radiation therapy
        Phototherapy for jaundice
        Hydrogen peroxide infusion
        Ozone
        Hyperbaric oxygen

Therapies utilizing harmful antioxidants:
        Too many to list

Stop the fatigue.
Stop staying tired.
Stop antioxidant overloading.
Stop protecting pathogens.
Stop sheltering cancer cells.
Stop antioxidant overkill!!

Ten great dietary supplement questions with 10 shocking answers:

1) Do the advertisers of dietary supplements repeatedly lie to us? Yes!

2) Does anyone regulate the ads of these advertisers? No!

3) Is the dietary supplement industry making $26 billion yearly? Yes!

4) Are their deceptive ads going to stop? No!

5) Are the misleading ads going to get any better? Of course not!

6) Do governmental agencies test any of the supplements for safety or effectiveness? No!

7) Do governmental agencies test any of the supplements for contaminants or purity? No!

8) Can the supplements claim to cure or diagnose any disease? No!

9) Can the supplements claim to prevent or treat any disease? No!

10) Other than a deficiency state, have supplements been scientifically proven to cure or reverse any disease at all? Nope, nada, zippo, none at all!

The secret to longevity is to keep breathing oxygen.
RMH 6-8-11

My epiphany of 4-4-11. I believe that the antioxidant overkill is doing the following: the over supply of electrons by the electron donating antioxidants are allowing the 4 electron reduction of ground state oxygen (O_2) to proceed to the final step, i.e., the formation of water. In doing so, this in effect "removes" the magically acting EMOD intermediates of superoxide, hydrogen peroxide, the hydroxyl radical, nitric oxide and peroxynitrite and "supplies" the non-reacting (non-protective) water to or within the milieu (intra- or extracellular). This, in effect, "quenches" the EMODs or ROS and it also prevents the protective action (messaging) of the reactive EMODs against pathogens and cancer. This is an entirely new paradigm. This is how it is happening and explains the electron donating nature of the antioxidants and the electron accepting nature of oxygen. This explains "how" the antioxidant overkill causes a harmful effect!!!!!

The antioxidant overload negates the beneficent actions of the intermediate EMODs. However, when the electron donating antioxidants are present in limited amounts, they serve as pre-oxidants or co-oxidants and form the active intermediates and reactive EMODs, after interacting with triplet oxygen. RMH

Finally, this explains the need for average amounts of antioxidants contained within a balanced nutritious diet, containing fresh fruits and vegetables. It also explains the failures of the antioxidant supplement studies, which were supplying an antioxidant overkill, thereby negating the protective EMOD effects against cancer and pathogens.

It has always puzzled me that antioxidants are "necessary" to form EMODs. In fact, this is why I referred to them as pre-oxidants or co-oxidants. The query for me was, "Then, how could the antioxidants be harmful?" Without them, ground state oxygen does not have an adequate source of available electrons to form the intermediate **EMODs**, i.e., the 1e (e, electron), 2e and 3e reduction products. But, with a sufficient amount of antioxidant electrons, oxygen can accept the electrons to form superoxide, hydrogen peroxide, the hydroxyl radical, nitric oxide and peroxynitrite, the active **EMOD** forms.

The basic redox chemistry is correct in that oxygen is the ultimate electron acceptor and antioxidants are the agent donating the electrons. This also explains the reason that transition metals, such as iron or copper, can also donate electrons to ground state oxygen and act as prooxidants. It is their contributions as electron donors that they are acting to form the protective prooxidant **EMOD** intermediates.

Part of the problem is that our diet and our environment supply us with adequate (and sometimes over supply us) with antioxidants. When we endeavor to "supplement" these sources, we over load the electron supply to oxygen and thus, it undergoes a 4 electron reduction to form water. **Wow!!!! This is way cool.**

Oxygen doesn't make you age.
It "allows" you to age.
Want proof?
Try aging without it!
R. M. Howes, M.D., Ph.D.
8/17/11

Note: It is beyond the scope of this book to review all of the antioxidant trials. Thus, the reader is referred to the vast literature on this subject.

Seven essential oxidative systems

Anyone who understands oxidative biochemistry readily knows that excessive antioxidants will interfere with or completely block crucial homeostatic and protective pathways in man.

Seven major systems utilize and need EMODs:

1) the immune system

2) cancer control

3) pathogen protection

4) energy production

5) wound healing

6) detoxification

7) cellular communication (cellular signaling)

The "7 oops"

I will refer to the unintended antioxidant interference with the seven essential prooxidative systems as the "7 oops." This implies that when excess antioxidants interfere with any or all of these pathways, the harmful unintended consequences are nonchalantly tossed off as an "oops." But, the deadly consequences are much more serious than that.

Please remember that the deadly unintended consequences of antioxidant overload are avoidable!

Mnemonic for the "7 oops" oxidative systems, "CC-WIPED": Cellular communication, Cancer protection, Wound healing, Immunity, Pathogen protection, Energy production and Detoxification.

Since antioxidants can interfere with or block any of these crucial systems, I question the need for antioxidant supplementation (except in cases of proven deficiencies or malabsorption syndromes), as I believe supplementation can actually decrease the effectiveness of any or all of these essential seven oxidative systems.

The scientific data backs up my assertions, which are the focus of my work.

ANTIOXIDANT OVERALL HARM

Safety is the overarching issue in drug development today.

In summary, scientific testing of some antioxidant study reports have selectively shown the following:

Antioxidants have increased mortality by as high as 17% and 19%.

Antioxidants have increased lung cancer by 18% and 28%, esophageal cancer deaths by 14% and 22.1%, breast cancer by 19%, hemorrhagic stroke deaths by 50%, ischemic heart disease by 11%, and cardiovascular disease by 18%.

Vitamin E increased risk of prostate cancer by 17%.

Antioxidants have increased prostate cancer deaths, elevated the risk of squamous cell carcinoma, doubled the risk of adenoma recurrence, increased the rate of second primary cancers, and increased recurrence of head and neck tumors.

Antioxidants increased the incidence of melanoma in women by 4 fold. (Hercberg et al, 2007, VITAL)

Patients taking an antioxidant were 1.65 times more likely to suffer a return of their original cancer.

Three major studies were stopped early due to unexpected harmful outcomes and adverse effects for study participants: ATBC, CARET and SELECT. (Heinonen et al, 1994, ATBC) (Omenn et al, 1996, CARET) (Lippman et al, 2009, SELECT) respectively.

Antioxidants have increased ischemic heart disease, deaths from fatal coronary heart disease, increased risk of nonfatal and fatal myocardial infarction, decreased platelet function, increased intima-to-media thickness, negated statin effects, increased risk of hospitalization for heart failure and hypertension, altered liver function tests, increased blood pressure, and increased blood loss after cardiac surgery.

Antioxidants have increased hemorrhagic stroke deaths as much as 22% to 50%, increased risk of subarachnoid hemorrhage 50% and increased risk of intracerebral hemorrhage 62% and increased risk of fatal subarachnoid hemorrhage 181%.

Antioxidants have increased wheezing, productive coughs, and risk of asthma.

In diabetics, antioxidants have increased pre-diabetic changes in glucose metabolism, increased severity of diabetic retinopathy, and increased blood pressure.

Antioxidants have increased preterm deliveries, premature rupture of membranes and low birth weight, increased gestational hypertension, increased risk of hospitalization, altered liver function tests, increased risk for severe preeclampsia, and fetal loss or perinatal death in women at risk for preeclampsia.

Antioxidants have increased risk of tuberculosis by 72% and pneumonia by 14%, indicating an altered immune system.

Antioxidants have adversely affected muscle performance and hampered endurance capacity.

Antioxidants increased risk of cataracts by 38% and by 56% in hormone replacement users, and increased risk of age-related macular degeneration (AMD).

Antioxidants increased the risk of hip fractures, damaged sperm DNA, increased epistaxis (nose bleed) and mother to child transfer of HIV.

Other than that....

Cancer related harmful effects of antioxidants: (new findings as of 10-29-11)

Antioxidants BHA and BHT increase carcinogenesis in animal studies.

The antioxidant, genistein, can cause chromosomal aberrations and DNA damage, in sperm and lymphocytes.
Genistein (an antioxidant) enhances growth of breast cancer cells in vitro.

Supplementation studies indicate soy may promote breast cancer development.

Combinations of antioxidants C and E may cause sperm damage.

Genistein (an antioxidant) induces DNA breaks in human tumor cell line and induced mitogenesis in mouse tumors.

Lycopene (an antioxidant) facilitated invasion of prostate cancer cells in vitro.

Selenium increased basal cell, squamous cell and total nonmelanoma skin cancer (NPC Trial).
Genistein (an antioxidant) enhanced tumor development of estrogen-dependent cells treated with carcinogens.

Genistein (an antioxidant) blocked the chemotherapy drug, tamoxifen, and attenuates its anti-tumor effect.

Vitamin E caused DNA damage in African-American men.

Excessive multivitamin use increased risk of fatal prostate cancers.

Vitamin E increased risk of oral premalignant lesions.

Genistein (an antioxidant) increased genomic instability of mouse lymphoma cells.
Genistein (an antioxidant) can reverse the cancer-inhibitory effect of anti-tumor agents.

Polymorphisms of the antioxidant enzyme, GPx1, increase risk of cancer.

Selenium (an antioxidant) can enhance mutagenesis and chromosomal abnormalities.

Genistein (an antioxidant) caused teratogenic effects in zebra fish embryos.

Alpha-tocopherol (vit E) increased adenocarcinomas of mammary glands in rats.

Carotenoids (an antioxidant) increased the risk of dying from cancer in women.

Genistein increased aromatase in human adrenocortical cancer in rats.

Neither the American Cancer Society nor the American Institute for Cancer Research recommend any dietary supplement for preventing cancer or cancer recurrence.

Other harmful effects of antioxidants:

Vitamin E and C slowed greyhound dogs.

Vitamin E made respiratory infections more severe.

Glutathione peroxidase (GPx1) interfered with insulin function and caused glucose intolerance.

Genistein produced a wide range of reproductive biological and behavioral defects in rats.

Vitamin C combined with grape seed extract increase systolic BP and diastolic BP.

Alpha-tocopherol caused an unexpected increase in cholesterol levels.

Thirteen percent (13.3%) of supplement users attributed adverse effects to multivitamins/multiminerals.

Alpha-tocopherol (and mixed tocopherols) increased systolic and diastolic BP and pulse pressure and heart rate, esp. in type 2 diabetes patients.

Vitamin A increased mother-to-infant risk of transmission of HIV.

Selenium increased risk of type 2 diabetes.

Post-exercise antioxidants negated good effects on lowering BP and vasodilation.

Antioxidants appear to hinder post-exercise recovery of muscle damage.

The casual use of vitamins C and E are not recommended for athletes.

Vitamin A increased risk of acute respiratory infection.

Vitamins A and C increase risk of gestational hypertension and low birth weights of neonates (newborns).

Bisphenol A (BPA, an antioxidant) decreased semen quality and increased sperm DNA damage.

Multivitamin/minerals caused third trimester women to experience preterm birth.

Selenium over use causes a wide range of effects, including fatigue and hair loss.

Soy products, isoflavones and genistein has implications for testicular malfunction in neonates.

Fats found in fish oil can block chemotherapy drugs in mice.

Taking supplements increased the risk of dying by 2.4% in women.

Vitamin E and beta-carotene increased risk of age-related macular degeneration.

BPA before birth negatively affected girl's behavior at age 3.

Use of multivitamins, B6, folic acid, magnesium, zinc, iron and copper increased risk of all-cause mortality.

Additionally, over 430 scientific studies have reported on the ineffectiveness of the antioxidants. They also indicate that unless there is a proven deficiency state, these antioxidants are unnecessary and dangerous. Further, the antioxidants in supplements do not work as effectively as those found in fresh fruits and vegetables.

ANTIOXIDANTS SHIELD CANCER CELLS

Also, we must keep in mind the fact that antioxidants protect cancer cells in vitro.

Human cancer cell types (27 human & 9 murine) shielded by antioxidants

If you are worried about cancer, just take a look at the human cell types that are protected by antioxidants from cell death in lab experiments.

Unbelievably, there are twenty seven (27) types of human cancer cell types and nine (9) murine cancer cell types that can be killed by EMODs and in which the killing can be blocked by antioxidants, thereby providing antioxidant protection and shielding of the cancer cells. Published data has shown that antioxidants blocked the killing of the following human and murine (rodent) cancer cell types by EMODs:

- **human breast cancer** (J. Nutr. 134, 2004) (Gundimeda et al, 1996) (Peralta et al, 2006) (Aykin-Burns et al, 2009) (Xiao et al, Mol Cancer Ther. 2006)

- **human prostate carcinoma** (Xiao et al, 2006) (Wu et al, 2005) (Singh et al, 2005) (Cho et al, 2005) (Milanesa et al, 2000)

- **human non-small cell lung cancer** (Ling et al, 2003) (Wu et al, 2006)

- **human colon adenocarcinoma** (Wenzel et al, 2005)

- **human colon cancer** (Wenzel et al, 2004) (Aykin-Burns et al, 2009)

- **human colorectal carcinoma** (Chen et al, 2004) (Gali-Muhtasib et al, 2008)

- **human ovarian cancer cells** (Pak et al, 2011)

- **human melanoma** (Marcin et al, 2005) (Okroj et al, 2006) (Nishikawa et al, 2004) (Grimm et al, 2011)

- **human metastatic melanoma** (Kirshner et al, 2008)

- **human head and neck cancer** (Mattson et al, 2009) (Simons et al, 2007)

- **human lymphoma** (J. Nutr. 134, 2004) (Mansat-De Mas et al, 1999)

- **human leukemia** (Hileman et al, 2004) (McKallip et al, 2006) (Hou et al, 2005) (Feng et al, 2007) (Yedjou et al, 2008) (Hiraoka et al, 1998)

- **human hepatoma** (Wu et al, 2004) (Wu, Ng, Lin, 2004)

- **human hepatocellular liver carcinoma** (Shimoda et al, 2003)

- **human pancreatic cancer** (Maehara et al, 2004)

- **human multiple myeloma** (Grad et al, 2001) (Ahmad et al, 1997) (Gupta et al, 2000) (Nakazato et al, 2005) (Isham et al, 2007)

- **Burkitt's lymphoma** (Ahmad et al, 1997) (Gupta et al, 2000) (Nakazato et al, 2005) (Ahmad et al, 1997)

- **human chronic lymphocytic leukemia** (Kay, 2006) (Chandra et al, 2003) (Shanafelt et al, 2005) (Mow et al, 2002) (Biswas S, et al, 2010)

- **human acute myeloid leukemia** (Kay, 2006) (Chandra et al, 2003) (Shanafelt et al, 2005) (Mow et al, 2002)

- **human promyelocytic leukemia** (Hou et al, 2005)

- **human erythromyeloid leukemia** (Wagner et al, 2000)

- **human epithelial cancer cells** (breast and colon) (Aykin-Burns et al, 2009)

- **human endometrial cancer** (Llobet et al, 2008)

- **human bladder cancer cells** (Miyajima et al, 1999)

- **human invasive bladder cancer** (Miyajima et al, 1999 - human bladder cancer KU-1 cell line)

- **human glioblastoma cells** (Lee et al, 2004)

- **human osteosarcoma** (Ahmad et al, 2005)

- **murine pheochromocytoma** (Jang, Surh, 2001)

- **murine retinoblastoma** (Salganik et al, 2000)

- **murine thymoma** (Tome et al, 2001)

- **murine lymphoma- six cell types** (Nathan et al, vol 153, 1981)

- **murine leukemia** (Wagner et al, 1996)

- **murine fibrosarcoma** (Teicher et al, 1994)

- **murine neuroblastoma** (Prasad et al, PNAS. 1979)

- **murine mammary cancer** (Bracke et al, 1999)

- **murine brain cancer** (Zeisel (2), 2004)

OTHER known human cancer cell types killed by EMODs

- **human prostate cancer cells:** androgen-independent human prostate cancer **PC-3 (Wt)** cells (Venkataraman et al, 2004), (Venkataraman et al, 2005),

- **human diploid leukemia cells: PLB-985** myeloid leukemia cells (Hiraoka et al, 1998)

- **human leukemia cells isolated from patients:** human monoblastic **ML-1 and lymphoblastoid T-cell Jurkat** lines (Pelicano et al, 2003) (McKallip et al, 2006) (Ahmad et al, 2003)

- **human colon cancer cells: HT-29** colon cancer cells (Malik et al, 2003)

Part of this list was compiled in 2009 and has been updated for this book. (Howes, Philica. Feb 7, 2009). **It is evident to many investigators that the in vitro apoptogenic agents function as prooxidants.** (Hail et al, 2008). Note: References for this list are available in my book, *Dangers of Excessive Antioxidants In Cancer Patients, 2011*.

Organizations not recommending antioxidant vitamins

Contrary to the common impression, major health organizations do not recommend the antioxidant vitamins A, C and E.

THE FOLLOWING LIST PROVIDES THE MAJOR MEDICAL AND SCIENTIFIC ORGANIZATIONS WHICH DO NOT RECOMMEND THE USE OF ANTIOXIDANT VITAMINS

The following either do not recommend antioxidant vitamins or have found inconclusive evidence of their benefit:

- **The U.S. Food and Drug Administration (FDA)**

- **The American Heart Association (AHA)**

- **The American Cancer Society (ACS)**

- **The National Cancer Institute (NCI)**

- **Institute of Medicine of the National Academies**

- **The American College of Cardiology**

- **The American College of Chest Physicians (ACCP)**

- **The American Diabetes Association**

- **The American Academy of Family Physicians**

- **Scientific Statement From the American Heart Association and the American Diabetes Association**

- **The American College of Cardiology/American Heart Association Task Force on Practice Guidelines**

- **United States Preventive Services Task Force (USPSTF)**

- The American Cancer Society Guidelines on Nutrition and Physical Activity for Cancer Prevention

- The Nutrition Committee of the American Heart Association Council on Nutrition, Physical Activity, and Metabolism

- The AHA Scientific Position of the American Heart Association

- The Canadian Task Force on Preventive Health Care (CTFPHC)

- Food and Nutrition Board, Institute of Medicine

- The Food and Nutrition Board of the National Academy of Sciences

- National Academy of Sciences

- The 2006 AHA Diet and Lifestyle Recommendations

- The Medical Letter

- The Oregon Health and Science University

- Food Standards Agency/ the British Nutrition Foundation (BNF)

- Quackwatch

- American College of Cardiology Foundation Task Force on Clinical Expert Consensus Documents

-
- National Institutes of Health State-of-the-Science Conference

- The American Heart Association Atherosclerosis, Hypertension, and Obesity in Youth Committee, Council of Cardiovascular Disease in the Young, With the Council on Cardiovascular Nursing

- The Physicians Health Study

-   **The 2008 VITAmins and Lifestyle (VITAL) study**

-   **The Physicians' Health Study II Randomized Controlled Trial**

-   **The Swedish Council of Technology Assessment**

-   **National Heart Foundation of Australia's Nutrition and Metabolism Advisory Committee**

Although their conclusions are not iron clad, many prestigious scientific organizations have concluded that,"taking antioxidant vitamins - such as vitamins A, C and E - serves no purpose, and in some cases could likely be harmful."

Such a list is rather astounding because broadcast media presents a never-ending cycle of advertisements pushing the wonders of antioxidants and antioxidant vitamins. One would assume that such advertisements would have the backing of major medical and scientific organizations, but that is not the case.

The above 32 conclusions or recommendations are apparently some of the best kept secrets in America, since antioxidants are being fortified or added to a wide spectrum of commercial products including foods, cosmetics, dermatologics, pet products, beverages, energy drinks, energy bars, fruits drinks, fruit juices, chewing gum, shampoos, etc. **Genetic engineers are hurriedly creating "super foods," which will be "antioxidant-rich."** (Howes R.M. 2009, Am J Cosm Surg)

It becomes readily apparent that maintaining sufficient EMOD levels can be extremely challenging.

As I have said many times, oxidation and reduction are flip sides of the same redox coin!

None of these systems are purely antioxidative or prooxidative in nature.

This study illustrates the difficulty in studying redox agents, many of which possess both antioxidative and prooxidative qualities.

ABOUT THE AUTHOR

Dr. Randolph M. Howes M.D., Ph.D.

Biographical sketch:

As a champion of the people, Dr. Howes anticipates and hopes for the active involvement of all connected parties (patients, caregivers, healthcare professionals, etc.) as an integral approach to educating consumers and the public about the potential dangers of excessive antioxidant-containing supplements.

Some people are born with a silver spoon in their mouth but Dr. Howes had to earn his. Even as a child, Dr. Howes could think with adult clarity. He could envision his future but it would require "decades of dedication" to make it a reality.

From childhood, Dr. Howes was motivated to become a medical doctor and scientist. Assuredly, having been born on a small strawberry farm in rural Louisiana, his journey to the top has proved to be arduous and demanding.

However, he was fortunate to acquire the confidence of Sister Elizabeth at St. Joseph's school and went on to gain the support of his high school speech teacher, Mrs. Iris Brann, who also had strong beliefs in his abilities and potential. Ultimately, with the help of his guitar and his singing ability, he defeated the star quarter back of the high school football team to become the president of the student body.

With the aid of a $25 dollar legislative scholarship, he went on to Southeastern Louisiana College (SLC). At SLC, he was selected for honors chemistry, made the Dean's list, worked at the Psychology Research Lab forty hours a week, maintained a premed study load, and was elected president of the Junior Class and the Interfraternity Council.

To earn badly needed funds, he played music on weekends in a small combo, The Three Blind Mice. Next, he matriculated to Tulane University School of Medicine.

His initial dream was to try to combine both medicine and science. In that regard, he began work as a technician with Dr. Andrew Schally at the Endocrine Polypeptide Lab in the isolation of thyrotropin releasing factor. This work led to a Nobel Prize for Dr. Schally.

Dr. Howes had been highly impressed with the enthusiasm of biochemist, Dr. Richard H. Steele, who accepted him as a doctoral candidate under his tutelage. Dr. Howes graduated in the top 10 of his class, won the Louisiana Pathology Association Award, was elected to the Sigma Xi honor fraternity and was the first in the history of Tulane to become a Doctor of Medicine and a Ph.D. in biochemistry concurrently.

Next, he was selected to pursue a career in surgery at the prestigious Johns Hopkins Hospital.

Unbelievably, at Dr. Howes' urging, he was allowed to operate his own research lab during his surgical internship and residency training while at Johns Hopkins Hospital. He worked hand in hand with the greats in American medicine and surgery.

Independently, he garnered grants, trained lab techs, wrote papers, slept on the cold floor, proudly served as a Captain in the U.S. Army Reserves Medical Corp and finished with board eligibility in both general and plastic surgery in an unheard of six year period.

In another first, he was appointed as an Adjunct Assistant Professor of Plastic Surgery at Johns Hopkins Hospital.

For decades, Dr. Howes gave unselfishly to pro bono medical missions in the Philippines and he holds the Ernesto Espaldon Chair as Professor of Plastic Surgery at the University of Santo Tomas.

Upon retirement from a career in cosmetic plastic surgery, he is living his dream of trying to revolutionize the treatment of cancer, heart disease, HIV/AIDS and malaria, with his in depth knowledge of the arcane biochemistry of oxygen metabolism. He is a work in progress! Dedicated and passionate, he is on a mission for mankind.

Dr. Howes invented the triple lumen venous catheter, which has been credited with helping save the lives of over 20 million critically ill patients worldwide. His catheter is the number one venous catheter in the world today and his name is well recognized in over 100 countries.

He has been recognized as a humanitarian, visionary, entrepreneur, singer, songwriter, inventor and author.

He received the Harper Award for innovative research from the American College for Advancement in Medicine, served as their keynote speaker and his peers refer to him as "a walking encyclopedia on oxygen metabolism."

He is a Dr. Norman Vincent Peale Unsung Hero award winner, which recognized his awesome versatility. Additionally, even though he is humble and does not like talking about it, he is a self made multi-millionaire.

He is currently doing extensive research on cures for cancer and heart disease and development of revolutionary treatment modalities. He has written 18 books over the past 5 years on the subject of oxygen metabolism, as it relates to protection from cancer, heart disease, diabetes, malaria, HIV/AIDS, Alzheimer's disease, aging and arthritis. He has written many scientific and medical papers and has lectured nationally and internationally. He has written over 500 medical letters to the editor on popular topics.

His research has shown that currently common antioxidant vitamins, such as vitamins A & E, (and vitamin C to a lesser extent) can be harmful and that oxygen free radicals protect us from bacterial, fungal and viral infections and they help to control cancer growth.

He has developed an effective, inexpensive singlet oxygen generating system, from orthomolecular agents, for the treatment of cancer and heart disease. He is passionate about his research and hopes to have his discoveries at the patient's bedside in his lifetime. Admittedly, this is an extremely ambitious goal.

There are over 10,000 pages in his magnum opus and at the Howes World Selective Library on Oxygen Metabolism. **Over 3,000 pages of his opus are available online in a searchable format www. iwillfindthecure.org** © 2011 by R.M. Howes

The scientific method demands that we change our beliefs or theories to fit the factual data. I believe that this applies directly to the Free Radi-Crap theory. Again, I say to you, "The free radical theory has fallen and so has the mitochondrial free radical theory of aging."

Companion Books of Prof. R. Howes, MD, PhD:

Howes, R. M. *U.T.O.P.I.A. - Unified Theory of Oxygen Participation in Aerobiosis.* © 2004. Free Radical Publishing Co. Kentwood, LA, available at www.iwillfindthecure.org.

Howes R. M. *The Medical and Scientific Significance of Oxygen Free Radical Metabolism.* © 2005. Free Radical Publishing Co. Kentwood, LA. USA. available at www.iwillfindthecure.org.

Howes, R. M. *Hydrogen Peroxide Monograph 1: Scientific, Medical and Biochemical Overview.* © 2006; Free Radical Publishing Co. USA. 200 pages. available at www.iwillfindthecure.org.

Howes, R. M. Monograph 2: *Antioxidant vitamins A, C & E: Equivocal Scientific Studies,* © 2006; Free Radical Publishing Co. USA. 171 pages. available at www.iwillfindthecure.org.

Howes, R. M. *Cardiovascular Disease and Oxygen Free Radical Mythology,* © 2006; Free Radical Publishing Co. USA. 308 pages. available at www.iwillfindthecure.org.

Howes, R. M. *Diabetes and Oxygen Free Radical Sophistry,* © 2006; Free Radical Publishing Co. USA. Free Radical Publishing Co. USA. 366 pages. available at www.iwillfindthecure.org.

Howes, R. M. *Reactive Oxygen Species Insufficiency (ROSI) as the Basis for Disease Allowance and Coexistence: Extraordinary Support for an Extraordinary Theory* Vol I, II & III. © 2008; 1564 pages. available at www.iwillfindthecure. org.

Howes, R. M. Volume I 501 pages #7 © 2008. Free Radical Publishing Co. USA.

Howes, R. M. Volume II 505 pages #8 © 2008. Free Radical Publishing Co. USA.

Howes, R. M. Volume III 562 pages #9 © 2008. Free Radical Publishing Co. USA.

Howes, R. M. *THE HOWES PAPERS* © 2009; Free Radical Publishing Co. USA. 211 pages

Howes R.M. *"COFFEE TABLE MUSINGS of the Da Vinci in COWBOY BOOTS"* Pithy Prose and Perspicacious Aphorisms. © 2009; 103 pages

Howes, R. M. Reactive Oxygen Species vs. Antioxidants:
"The Oxypocalypse" or
"The war that never was" © 2010; Free Radical Publishing Co. USA. 550 pages. available at www.iwillfindthecure.org.

Howes R.M. *Death in Small Doses?:*
Antioxidant Vitamins A, C & E in the 21st Century
Book One: *A Health Impact Statement For The Layman*
© 2010; Trafford Publishing. Indianapolis, USA. 90 pages

Howes R.M. *Antioxidant Vitamins are Making A Killing;*
Antioxidant Vitamins A, C & E in the 21st Century
Book Two: *A Health Impact Statement For The Medical Scientist*
© 2010; 184 pages

- **Death In Small Doses? Trafford Publishing, © 2010**

- **Antioxidant Overkill, CreateSpace and Free Radical Publishing, © 2011**

- **Dangers of Excessive Antioxidants in Cancer Patients, CreateSpace and Free Radical Publishing, © 2011**

- **Heart Disease and Antioxidant Failures, CreateSpace and Free Radical Publishing, © 2011**

- **Antioxidant Failures and Dangers, CreateSpace and Free Radical Publishing, © 2011**

- **Anti-Aging Anti-oxidant Scams, CreateSpace and Free Radical Publishing, © 2011**

- **Sports, Athletes, Exercise Facts and Antioxidant Myths, CreateSpace and Free Radical Publishing, © 2011**

- **Alzheimer's Disease: Forget Antioxidants and Supplements, CreateSpace and Free Radical Publishing, © 2012**

- **Sex, Performance, Reproduction, Naked Radicals And Antioxidants, CreateSpace and Free Radical Publishing, © 2012**

- **Antioxidants Linked To Deadly Unintended Consequences, CreateSpace and Free Radical Publishing, © 2013**

- **U.T.O.P.I.A.: Unified Theory of Oxygen Participation In Aerobiosis, CreateSpace and Free Radical Publishing,** © 2014, revised

- **Hydrogen Peroxide: A Health, Homeostatic and Protective Essentiality, CreateSpace and Free Radical Publishing,** © 2014

- **Reactive Oxygen Species vs. Antioxidants: The Oxypocalypse or The War That Never Was, CreateSpace and Free Radical Publishing,** © 2014

- **Diabetes and Oxygen Free Radical Sophistry, CreateSpace and Free Radical Publishing,** © 2014, revised

- **FISH OIL (Omega3 fatty acids): Facts, Fantasies & Failures. CreateSpace and Free Radical Publishing,** © 2014

-**Vitamin D: Benefits & False claims. CreateSpace and Free Radical Publishing,** © 2014

- **Chocolate & Red Wine Antioxidants (Polyphenols, Flavonoids & Resveratrol): Facts vs. Falsehoods. CreateSpace and Free Radical Publishing,** © 2014)

All books available at www.amazon.com; www.barnesandnobles.com; www.booksamillion.com.

Companion Papers of Prof. R. Howes, MD, PhD:

Dr. Howes has authored over 450 medical publications in health related editorials.

Citation: R. Howes: Mythology of Antioxidant Vitamins?. *The Journal of Evidence-Based Alternative and Complimentary Medicine.* April, 2011. 16(2): 149-189.

Citation: R. Howes: Cancer Therapy: A Review with Scientific Validation for the Role of Electronically Modified Oxygen Derivatives in Oncologic Treatment Modalities. *The Internet Journal of Alternative Medicine.* 2010 Volume 8 Number 1.

Citation: R. Howes: Hydrogen Peroxide: A review of a scientifically verifiable omnipresent ubiquitous essentiality of obligate, aerobic, carbon-based life forms. *The Internet Journal of Plastic Surgery.* 2010 Volume 7 Number 1.

Howes M.D., PhD., R. (2009). Dangers of Antioxidants in Cancer Patients: A Review. *PHILICA.COM Article number 153.* Published 7th February, 2009. (20 pages)

Howes M.D., PhD., R. (2008). Aging and anti-aging claims: a review on antioxidant vitamins A, C & E. *PHILICA.COM Article number 116.* Published on 12th January, 2008. (16 pages)

Howes M.D., PhD., R. (2007). Sleep: An original "radical" proposal. *PHILICA.COM Observation number 42.* Published on 5th October, 2007. (1 page)

Howes M.D., PhD., R. (2007). Antioxidant Vitamins A, C & E: Death in Small Doses and Legal Liability? *PHILICA.COM Article number 89.* Published on 5th April, 2007. (23 pages)

Howes M.D., PhD., R. (2007). Cancer, Apoptosis and Reactive Oxygen Species: A New Paradigm. *PHILICA.COM Article number 86.* Published on 26th February, 2007. (11 pages)

Howes M.D., PhD., R. (2007). Antioxidant Vitamins A, C and E: Assessing Potential for Harm. *PHILICA.COM Article number 83.* Published on 15th February, 2007. (14 pages)

Howes M.D., PhD., R. (2007). The Consequent Downfall of the Free Radical Theory. *PHILICA.COM Article number 75.* Published on 22nd January, 2007. (9 pages)

Howes, R.M.: "The Free Radical Fantasy," The Annals of New York Academy of Sciences, 2006, Vol. 1067, pp. 22-26.

(Howes, 2005) (Howes, R.M. Tumoricidal Activity of An Injectable Singlet Oxygen System Generated From Physiological Agents: The Howes Singlet Oxygen Cancer Therapy System). In The Medical and Scientific Significance of Oxygen Free Radical Metabolism. © 2005. Free Radical Publishing Co. Kentwood, LA. pp. 893-912).

(Howes, Farber, 2005) (Howes, R.M. and Farber, G. Tumoricidal Activity of the Howes Singlet Oxygen Delivery System in Human Basal Cell Carcinoma. In The Medical and Scientific Significance of Oxygen Free Radical Metabolism. © 2005. Free Radical Publishing Co. Kentwood, LA. pp. 883-892).

(Howes et al, 1977) (Howes, R.M., Steele, R.H. and Hoopes, J.E., The role of Electronic excitation states in collagen biosynthesis, Persp. In Biol. And Med., Summer 1977, 20; 4:539-544).

(Howes, Steele, 1976) (Howes, R.M., Steele, R.H. and Hoopes, J.E., Peroxide induced Chemiluminescence in an in vitro proline hydroxylation system, 1976, 8; 1:77-84).

(Howes et al, 1976) (Howes, R. M., Allen, R.C., Su, C.T. and Hoopes, J.E., Altered polymorphonuclear leukocyte bioenergetics in patients with thermal injury, the Surgical Forum, 1976, 27:558-560).

(Howes, Steele, 1972) (Howes, R.M. and Steele, R.H., Microsomal chemiluminescence induced by NADPH and its relation to aryl-hydroxylations, Res Commun. Chem. Path. Pharmacol., March 1972, 3; 2:349-357).

(Howes, Steele, 1971) (Howes, R. M. and Steele, R. H., Microsomal chemiluminescence induced by NADPH and its relation to lipid peroxidation, Res. Commun. Chem. Path. Pharmacol., July-Sept. 1971, 2; 4 & 5:619-626).

**I despise precious time wasted,
for it alone, is the unfinished canvas
displaying the portrait of my life.
R. M. Howes, M.D., Ph.D.
9/7/09**

"**We are what we repeatedly do. Excellence then, is not an act, but a habit.**" ~**Aristotle**

OTHER BOOKS

PUBLISHED: Partial list. The Fire Eaters, Molding your own destiny more easily, Carnivore Press, © **1982**

Uplift, The Answer Book to your plastic and cosmetic surgery questions, Carnivore Press, © 1986

The Pundit Speaks, vol. I. An Anthology of Neoclassical Poetic Philosophy, Carnivore Press, © 1990

The Pundit Speaks, Volume II, An Anthology of Neoclassical Poetic Philosophy, Free Radical Press, © 1994

The Pundit Speaks, Volume III, An Anthology of Neoclassical Poetic Philosophy, Free Radical Press, © 1996

The Pundit Speaks, Volume IV, An Anthology of Neoclassical Poetic Philosophy, Free Radical Press, © 2000

The Fable of the Chocolate Covered Strawberry Coloring Book, Free Radical Press, © 2001

The Pundit Speaks, Volume IV, An Anthology of Neoclassical Poetic Philosophy, Free Radical Press, © 2003

The Pundit Speaks, Volume V, An Anthology of Neoclassical Poetic Philosophy, Trafford Publishing, © 2009

Coffee Table Musings of The DaVinci In Cowboy Boots, Trafford Publishing, © 2010

Available at: www.philica.com
www.medi.philica.com
www.iwillfindthecure.org
www.amazon.com

DOC
R$_x$ANDOLPH
HOWES

RAD!CAL

**"Future's shape is sculpted by the
persistent kneading hands of
the impossible dreamer."**
R. M. Howes, M.D., Ph.D.
5/2/04

References

(Ahmadvand, Ghaseme-Dehnoo, 2014) (Ahmadvand H, Ghasemi-Dehnoo M. Antiatherogenic, hepatoprotective, and hypolipidemic effects of coenzyme Q10 in alloxan-induced type 1 diabetic rats. ARYA Atheroscler. 2014 Jul;10(4):192-8)

(Ahmet et al, 2009) (Ahmet I, et al. Blueberry-enriched diet protects rat heart from ischemic damage. PLoS One. (2009)

(Aires et al, 2012) (Aires DJ, et al. Potentiation of dietary restriction-induced lifespan extension by polyphenols. Biochim Biophys Acta. (2012)

(Allen et al, 2003) (Allen CM, Schwartz SJ, Craft NE, Giovannucci EL, De Groff VL, Clinton SK. Changes in plasma and oral mucosal lycopene isomer concentrations in healthy adults consuming standard servings of processed tomato products. Nutrition and Cancer. 2003;47(1):48–56)

(Andres-Lacueva et al, 2005) (Andres-Lacueva C, et al. Anthocyanins in aged blueberry-fed rats are found centrally and may enhance memory. Nutr Neurosci. (2005)

(Anonymous, 2000) (Anonymous, Dietary reference intakes for vitamin C, vitamin E, selenium, and carotenoids, Beta-carotene and other carotenoids. Washinton, D.C: National Academies Press; 2000)

(Antartani, Ashok, 2011) (Antartani R, Ashok K. Effect of lycopene in prevention of preeclampsia in high risk pregnant women. J Turk Ger Gynecol Assoc. 2011; 12(1):35-38)

(Aquilano et al, 2008) (Aquilano K, Baldelli S, Rotilio G, Ciriolo MR. Role of nitric oxide synthases in Parkinson's disease: a review on the antioxidant and anti-inflammatory activity of polyphenols. Neurochem Res. 2008;33:2416–2426)

(Arab, Elsahoff, 2009) (Arab L, Liu W, Elashoff D. Green and black tea consumption and risk of stroke. a meta-analysis. Stroke. 2009;40:1786–92)

(Arts, Hollman, 2005) (Arts ICW, Hollman PCH. Polyphenols and disease risk in epidemiologic studies. Am J Clin Nutr. 2005;81:317–325)

(Athar et al, 2007) (Athar M, Back JH, Tang X, Kim KH, Kopelovich L, Bickers DR, Kim AL. Resveratrol: a review of preclinical studies for human cancer prevention. Toxicol Appl Pharmacol. 2007;224:274–283)

(Aviram et al., 2000) (Aviram, M., Dornfeld, L., Rosenblat, M., Volkova, N., Hayek, T., Presser, D., Attias, J, Liker, H., Gaitini, D., Nitecki, S. Pomegranate juice consumption for 3 years by patients with carotid artery stenosis reduces common carotid intima-media thickness, blood pressure and LDL oxidation. Clin Nutr. 2004 Jun; 23(3): 423-33)

(Bachman et al, 2008) (Bachman JL, Reedy J, Subar AF, Krebs-Smith SM. Sources of food group intakes among the US population, 2001–2002. J Am Diet Assoc. 2008;108:804–814)

(Bagchi et al, 1997) (Bagchi D, Garg A, Krohn RL et al. Oxygen free radical scavenging abilities of Vitamin C and E' and a grape seed proanthocyanidin extract in vitro. Res Commun Mol Pathol Pharmacol 1997; 95: 179-89)

(Basu et al, 2010) (Arpita Basu, Michael Rhone, and Timothy J Lyons. Berries: emerging impact on cardiovascular health. Nutr Rev. Mar 2010; 68(3): 168–177)

(Biddle, et al, 2013) (Biddle M, et al. Higher dietary lycopene intake is associated with longer cardiac event-free survival in patients with heart failure. Eur J Cardiovasc Nurs. Aug 2013; 12(4): 377-384)

(Bingul et al, 2013) (Bingül I, et al. Effect of blueberry pretreatment on diethylnitrosamine-induced oxidative stress and liver injury in rats. Environ Toxicol Pharmacol. (2013)

(Bishayee, 2009) (Bishayee A. Cancer prevention and treatment with resveratrol: from rodent studies to clinical trials. Cancer Prevention Research 2:409-418, 2009)

(Bjelakovic et al, 2008) (Bjelakovic G, Nikolova D, Gluud LL, Simonetti RG, Gluud C. Cochrane Database Syst Rev.2008: CD007176)

(Block et al, 1992) (Block G, Patterson B, Subar A. Fruit, vegetables, and cancer prevention: A review of the epidemiological evidence. Nutrition and Cancer. 1992;18(1):1–29)

(Boehm et al, 2009) (Boehm et al. Green tea (Camellia sinensis) for the prevention of cancer. Cochrane Database Syst Rev. 2009 Jul 8;(3): CD005004)

(Bogsrud et al, 2013) (No effect of combined coenzyme Q10 and selenium supplementation on atorvastatin-induced myopathy. Bogsrud MP, Langslet G, Ose L, Arnesen KE, Sm Stuen MC, Malt UF, Woldseth B, Retterstøl K. Scand Cardiovasc J. 2013 Apr;47(2):80-7)

(Bohm, Bitsch, 1999) (Bohm V, Bitsch R. Intestinal absorption of lycopene from different matrices and interactions to other carotenoids, the lipid status, and the antioxidant capacity of human plasma. European Journal of Nutrition. 1999;38(3):118–125)

(Bohm, 2012) (Böhm V. Lycopene and heart health. Mol Nutr Food Res. 2012 Feb;56(2):296-303. doi: 10.1002/mnfr.769)

(Boileau et al, 2003) (Boileau TW, Liao Z, Kim S, Lemeshow S, Erdman JW, Jr, Clinton SK. Prostate carcinogenesis in n-methyl-n-nitrosourea (nmu)-testosterone-treated rats fed tomato powder, lycopene, or energy-restricted diets. Journal of the National Cancer Institute. 2003;95(21):1578–1586)

(Bom et al, 2014) (Jenifer Bom, Patrícia Gunutzmann, Elizabeth C. Pérez Hurtado, Jussara M. R. Maragno-Correa, Silvia Regina Kleeb, and Maria Anete Lallo Long-Term Treatment with Aqueous Garlic and/or Tomato Suspensions Decreases Ehrlich Ascites Tumors. Evid Based Complement Alternat Med. 2014; 2014: 381649)

(Bookstaver et al, 2012) (Effect of coenzyme Q10 supplementation on statin-induced myalgias. Bookstaver DA, Burkhalter NA, Hatzigeorgiou C. Am J Cardiol. 2012 Aug 15;110(4):526-9. doi: 10.1016/j.amjcard.2012.04.026. Epub 2012 May 18)

(Borges et al, 2010) (Borges G, et al. Identification of flavonoid and phenolic antioxidants in black currants, blueberries, raspberries, red currants, and cranberries. J Agric Food Chem. (2010)

(Bosetti et al, 2004) (Bosetti C, Talamini R, Montella M, Negri E, Conti E, Franceschi S, La Vecchia C. Int J Cancer.2004;112:689–692)

(Bowen et al, 2002) (Bowen P, Chen L, Stacewicz-Sapuntzakis M, Duncan C, Sharifi R, Ghosh L, et al. Tomato sauce supplementation and prostate cancer: lycopene accumulation and modulation of biomarkers of carcinogenesis. Experimental Biology and Medicine. 2002;227(10):886–893)

(Campbell et al, 2004) (Campbell JK, Canene-Adams K, Lindshield BL, Boileau TW, Clinton SK, Erdman JW Jr. Tomato phytochemicals and prostate cancer risk. J Nutr. 2004; 134:3486S-3492S)

(Canene-Adams et al, 2007) (Canene-Adams K, Lindshield BL, Wang S, Jeffery EH, Clinton SK, Erdman JW., Jr Combinations of tomato and broccoli enhance antitumor activity in dunning r3327-h prostate adenocarcinomas. Cancer Research. 2007;67(2):836–843)

(Cao, Prior, 1998) (G. Cao and R.L. Prior Comparison of different analytical methods for assessing total antioxidant capacity of human serum. Guohua Cao and Ronald L. Prior. Clinical Chemistry June 1998, 44 (6): 1309-1315)

(Cao, Cao, 1999) (Cao Y, Cao R. Angiogenesis inhibited by drinking tea. Nature1999;398:381)

(Carmen-Ramirez-Tortosa et al, 2004) (Carmen Ramirez-Tortosa M, et al. Oxidative stress status in an institutionalised elderly group after the intake of a phenolic-rich dessert. Br J Nutr. (2004)

(Cassidy et al, 2013) (Cassidy A, et al. High anthocyanin intake is associated with a reduced risk of myocardial infarction in young and middle-aged women. Circulation. (2013)

(Chalabi et al, 2006) (Chalabi N, Delort L, Le Corre L, Satih S, Bignon YJ, Bernard-Gallon D. Gene signature of breast cancer cell lines treated with lycopene. Pharmacogenomics. 2006;7(5):663–672)

(Chalabi, Delort et al, 2006) (Chalabi N, Delort L, Le Corre L, Satih S, Bignon YJ, Bernard-Gallon D. Gene signature of breast cancer cell lines treated with lycopene. Pharmacogenomics. 2006;7(5):663–672)

(Chalabi et al, 2007) (Chalabi N, Delort L, Satih S, Dechelotte P, Bignon YJ, Bernard-Gallon DJ. Immunohistochemical expression of raralpha, rarbeta, and cx43 in breast tumor cell lines after treatment with lycopene and correlation with rt-qpcr. The Journal of Histochemistry and Cytochemistry. 2007;55(9):877–883)

(Chalabi et al, 2007) (Chalabi N, Delort L, Satih S, Dechelotte P, Bignon YJ, Bernard-Gallon DJ. Immunohistochemical expression of raralpha, rarbeta, and cx43 in breast tumor cell lines after treatment with lycopene and correlation with rt-qpcr. The Journal of Histochemistry and Cytochemistry. 2007;55(9):877–883)

(Chandra et al, 2007) (Chandra RV, Prabhuji ML, Roopa DA, et al. Efficacy of lycopene in the treatment of gingivitis: a randomised, placebo-controlled clinical trial. Oral Health Prev Dent. 2007;5:327-336)

(Chang et al, 2005) (Chang S, Erdman JW, Jr, Clinton SK, Vadiveloo M, Strom SS, Yamamura Y, Duphorne CM, Spitz MR, Amos CI, Contois JH, Gu X, Babaian RJ, Scardino PT, Hursting SD. Nutr Cancer. 2005;53:127–134)

(Charge, Rudnicki, 2004) (Charge SBP, Rudnicki MA: Cellular and molecular regulation of muscle regeneration.

Physiol Rev 2004, 84(1):209-238)

(Chun et al, 2008) (Chun OK, Chung SJ, Claycombe KJ, Song WO. Serum C-reactive protein concentrations are inversely associated with dietary flavonoid intake in U.S. adults. J Nutr. 2008;138:753–760)

(Clark et al, 2006) (Clark PE, Hall MC, Borden LS Jr, et al. Phase I-II prospective dose-escalating trial of lycopene in patients with biochemical relapse of prostate cancer after definitive local therapy. Urology.2006;67:1257-1261)

(Clegg et al, 2011) (Clegg ME, et al. The addition of raspberries and blueberries to a starch-based food does not alter the glycaemic response. Br J Nutr. (2011)

(Clifford, 2000) (Clifford MN. Chlorogenic acids and other cinnamates. Nature, occurrence, dietary burden, absorption and metabolism. J Sci Food Agric. 2000;80:1033–1043)

(Clinical Trial.gov) (ClinicalTrials.gov NCT00920556 A Clinical Study to Assess the Safety and Activity of SRT501 Alone or in Combination With Bortezomib in Patients With Multiple Myeloma)

(Coban et al, 2013) (Çoban J, et al. Effect of blueberry feeding on lipids and oxidative stress in the serum, liver and aorta of Guinea pigs fed on a high-cholesterol diet. Biosci Biotechnol Biochem. (2013)

(Cohen et al, 1999) (Cohen, L.A., Zhao, Z., Pittman, B. and Khachik, F. (1999) Effect of dietary lycopene on N-methylnitrosourea-induced mammary tumorigenesis. Nutr. Cancer, 34, 153–159)

(Cohn et al, 2004) (Cohn W, Thurmann P, Tenter U, Aebischer C, Schierle J, Schalch W. Eur J Nutr. 2004;43:304–312)

(Comstock et al, 1991) (Comstock GW, Helzlsouer KJ, Bush TL. Am J Clin Nutr. 1991;53:260S–264S)

(Corder et al, 2006) (Corder R, Mullen W, Khan NQ, Marks SC, Wood EG, Carrier MJ, Crozier A (November 2006). "Oenology: red wine procyanidins and vascular health". Nature 444 (7119): 566)

(Coultrap et al, 2008) (Coultrap SJ, Bickford PC, Browning MD. Blueberry-enriched diet ameliorates age-related declines in NMDA receptor-dependent LTP. Age (Dordr). (2008)

(Crews et al, 2008) (Crews WD Jr, Harrison DW, Wright JW. A double-blind, placebo-controlled, randomized trial of the effects of dark chocolate and cocoa on variables associated with neuropsychological functioning and cardiovascular health: clinical findings from a sample of healthy, cognitively intact older adults. Am J Clin Nutr. 2008 Apr;87(4):872-80)

(Cui et al, 2008) (Cui Y, Shikany JM, Liu S, Shagufta Y, Rohan TE. Am J Clin Nutr. 2008;87:1009–1018)

(Davies, Hochstein, 1982) (Davies KJ, Hochstein P. Ubisemiquinone radicals in liver: implications for a mitochondrial Q cycle in vivo. Biochemical and biophysical research communications. 1982 Aug 31;107(4):1292-9)

(DeFuria et al, 2009) (DeFuria J, Bennett G, Strissel KJ, et al. Dietary blueberry attenuates whole-body insulin resistance in high fat-fed mice by reducing adipocyte death and its inflammatory sequelae. J Nutr. 2009;139:1510–1516)

(De Vera et al, 2008) (De Vera, Mary; Rahman, M. Mushfiqur; Rankin, James; Kopec, Jacek; Gao, Xiang; Choi, Hyon (2008). "Gout and the risk of Parkinson's disease: A cohort study". Arthritis & Rheumatism 59 (11): 1549–54)

(Del Bo et al, 2013) (Del Bo C, et al. A single portion of blueberry (Vaccinium corymbosum L) improves protection against DNA damage but not vascular function in healthy male volunteers. Nutr Res. (2013)

(Di Mascio et al, 1989) (Di Mascio P, Kaiser S, Sies H. Arch Biochem Biophys. 1989;274:532–538)

(Ding et al, 2006) (Ding M, Feng R, Wang SY, Bowman L, Lu Y, Qian Y, Castranova V, Jiang BH, Shi X. Cyanidin-3-glucoside, a natural product derived from blackberry, exhibits chemopreventive and chemotherapeutic activity. J Biol Chem. 2006;281(25):17359–17368)

(Ding et al, 2008) (Ding E, Hutfless S, Ding X, et al. Chocolate and prevention of cardiovascular disease: a systematic review. Nutrition &

Metabolism. 2006;3:2. Available at: http://www.pubmedcentral.nih.gov/ articlerender.fcgi?artid=1360667. Accessed November 5, 2008)

(Doyle et al, 2006) (Doyle C, Kushi LH, Byers T, et al. The 2006 Nutrition, Physical Activity and Cancer Survivorship Advisory Committee. American Cancer Society. Nutrition and physical activity during and after cancer treatment: an American Cancer Society guide for informed choices. CA Cancer J Clin. 2006;56:323-353)

(Dubick, Omaye, 2001) (Dubick MA, Omaye ST. Evidence for grape, wine and tea polyphenols as modulators of atherosclerosis and ischemic heart disease in humans. J Nutraceut Functional & Med Foods. 2001;3:67–93)

(Durairajanayagam et al, 2014) (Durairajanayagam D, Agarwal A, Ong C, Prashast P. Lycopene and male infertility. Asian J Androl. 2014 doi: 10.4103/1008-682X126384. In press)

(Duran-Prado et al, 2014) (Durán-Prado M, Frontiñán J, Santiago-Mora R, Peinado JR, Parrado-Fernández C, Gómez-Almagro MV, Moreno M, López-Domínguez JA, Villalba JM, Alcaín FJ. Coenzyme Q10 protects human endothelial cells from □-amyloid uptake and oxidative stress-induced injury. PLoS One. 2014 Oct 1;9(10): e109223. doi: 10.1371/ journal.pone.0109223. eCollection 2014)

(EFSA, 2010) (EFSA Panel on Dietetic Products, Nutrition and Allergies (2010). "Scientific Opinion on the substantiation of health claims related to various food(s)/food constituent(s) and protection of cells from premature aging, antioxidant activity, antioxidant content and antioxidant properties, and protection of DNA, proteins and lipids from oxidative damage pursuant to Article 13(1) of Regulation (EC) No 1924/2006". EFSA Journal 8 (2): 1489)

(Eliassen et al, 2012) (Eliassen AH, Hendrickson SJ, Brinton LA, Buring JE, Campos H, Dai Q, Dorgan JF, Franke AA, Gao YT, Goodman MT, Hallmans G, Helzlsouer KJ, Hoffman-Bolton J, Hulten K, Sesso HD, Sowell AL, Tamimi RM, Toniolo P, Wilkens LR, Winkvist A, Zeleniuch-Jacquotte A, Zheng W, Hankinson SE. J Natl Cancer Inst. 2012;104:1905–1916)

(Elks et al, 2011) (Elks CM, et al. A blueberry-enriched diet attenuates nephropathy in a rat model of hypertension via reduction in oxidative stress. PLoS One. (2011)

(Ellinger et al, 2009) (Ellinger S, Ellinger J, Müller SC, Stehle P. Tomatoes and lycopene in prevention and therapy--is there an evidence for prostate diseases? Aktuelle Urol. 2009 Jan;40(1):37-43. doi: 10.1055/s-2008-1077031. Epub 2009 Jan 28)

(Engler et al, 2004) (Engler MB, Engler MM, Chen CY et al. Flavonoid-rich dark chocolate improves endothelial function and increases plasma epicatechin concentrations in healthy adults. J Am Coll Nutr 2004; 23: 197-204)

(Erdman, Ford, Lindshield, 2008) (Erdman JW Jr, Ford NA, Lindshield BL. Are the health attributes of lycopene related to its antioxidant function? Arch Biochem Biophys. 2009 Mar 15;483(2):229-35. doi: 10.1016/j. abb.2008.10.022. Epub 2008 Nov 1)

(Erlund et al, 2008) (Erlund I, Koli R, Alfthan G, et al. Favorable effects of berry consumption on platelet function, blood pressure, and HDL cholesterol. Am J Clin Nutr. 2008;87:323–331)

(Etminan et al, 2004) (Etminan M, Takkouche B, Caamano-Isorna F. Cancer Epidemiol Biomarkers Prev. 2004;13:340–345)

(EU register, 2012) (EU Register of nutrition and health claims made on foods. http://ec.europa.eu/nuhclaims/?/ accessed May 01 2012)

(FDA, 2008) (Guidance for Industry, Food Labeling; Nutrient Content Claims; Definition for "High Potency" and Definition for "Antioxidant" for Use in Nutrient Content Claims for Dietary Supplements and Conventional Foods U.S. Department of Health and Human Services, Food and Drug Administration, Center for Food Safety and Applied Nutrition, June 2008)

(FDA, 2013) ("FDA approved drug products". US Food and Drug Administration. Retrieved 8 November 2013) ("Health Claims Meeting Significant Scientific Agreement". US Food and Drug Administration. Retrieved 8 November 2013)

(Falk et al, 2995) (Falk B, Gorev R, Zigel L, et al. Effect of lycopene supplementation on lung function after exercise in young athletes who complain of exercise-induced bronchoconstriction symptoms. Ann Allergy Asthma Immunol. 2005;94:480-485)

(Fedacko et al, 2013) (Coenzyme Q(10) and selenium in statin-associated myopathy treatment. Fedacko J, Pella D, Fedackova P, Hänninen O, Tuomainen P, Jarcuska P, Lopuchovsky T, Jedlickova L, Merkovska L, Littarru GP. Can J Physiol Pharmacol. 2013 Feb;91(2):165-70)

(Finkel and Holbrook, 2000) (Finkel T, Holbrook NJ. Oxidants, oxidative stress and the biology of ageing. Nature. 2000;408(6809):239–247)

(Flowers et al, 2014) (Flowers N, Hartley L, Todkill D, Stranges S, Rees K. Co-enzyme Q10 supplementation for the primary prevention of cardiovascular disease. Cochrane Database Syst Rev. 2014 Dec 4;12: CD010405)

(Gajendragadkar et al, 2014) (Gajendragadkar PR, Hubsch A, Mäki-Petäjä KM, Serg M, Wilkinson IB, Cheriyan J. Effects of oral lycopene supplementation on vascular function in patients with cardiovascular disease and healthy volunteers: a randomised controlled trial. PLoS One. 2014 Jun 9;9(6): e99070. doi: 10.1371/journal.pone.0099070. eCollection 2014)

(Gao et al, 2011) (Gao L, Mao Q, Cao J, Wang Y, Zhou X, Fan L. Effects of coenzyme Q10 on vascular endothelial function in humans: a meta-analysis of randomized controlled trials. Atherosclerosis. 2012 Apr;221(2):311-6. doi: 10.1016/j.atherosclerosis.2011.10.027. Epub 2011 Oct 25)

(Gaudet et al, 2004) (Gaudet MM, Britton JA, Kabat GC, Steck-Scott S, Eng SM, Teitelbaum SL, Terry MB, Neugut AI, Gammon MD. Cancer Epidemiol Biomarkers Prev. 2004;13:1485–1494)

(Geleijnse, Hollman, 2008) (Geleijnse JM, Hollman PCH. Flavonoids and cardiovascular health: which compounds, what mechanisms? Am J Clin Nutr. 2008;88:12–3)

(Giovannucci et al, 1995) (Giovannucci E, Ascherio A, Rimm EB, Stampfer MJ, Colditz GA, Willett WC. Intake of carotenoids and retinol in relation to risk of prostate cancer. Journal of the National Cancer Institute. 1995;87(23):1767–1776)

(Giovannucci, 1999) (Giovannucci E. Tomatoes, tomato-based products, lycopene, and cancer: Review of the epidemiologic literature. Journal of the National Cancer Institute. 1999;91(4):317–331)

(Giovannucci, 2005) (Giovannucci E. Tomato products, lycopene, and prostate cancer: A review of the epidemiological literature. The Journal of Nutrition. 2005;135(8):2030S–2031S)

(Giovannucci, 2007) (Giovannucci E. Does prostate-specific antigen screening influence the results of studies of tomatoes, lycopene, and prostate cancer risk? Journal of the National Cancer Institute. 2007.99:1060-1062)

(Gleimann et al, 2013) (Gliemann L, Schmidt JF, Olesen J, Biensø RS, Peronard SL, Grandjean SU, Mortensen SP, Nyberg M, Bangsbo J, Pilegaard H, Hellsten Y. Resveratrol blunts the positive effects of exercise training on cardiovascular health in aged men. J Physiol. 2013 Oct 15;591(Pt 20):5047-59)

(Goldfarb et al, 2011) (Goldfarb AH, Garten RS, Cho C, Chee PD, Chambers LA: Effects of a fruit/berry/vegetable supplement on muscle function and oxidative stress. Med Sci Sports Exerc 2011,43(3):501-508)

(Gonzalez, et al, 2013) (González CA, Sala N, Rokkas T (2013). "Gastric cancer: epidemiologic aspects". Helicobacter 18 (Supplement 1): 34–38) (Woo, Kim, 2013) (Woo HD, Kim J (2013). "Dietary flavonoid intake and smoking-related cancer risk: a meta-analysis". PLoS One 8 (9): e75604)

(Goodman et al, 2003) (Goodman GE, Schaffer S, Omenn GS, Chen C, King I. Cancer Epidemiol Biomarkers Prev.2003;12:518–526)

(Goodman et al,2006) (Goodman M,Bostick RM,Ward KC,et al.Lycopene intake and prostate cancer risk: effect modification by plasma antioxidants and the XRCC1 genotype. Nutrition & Cancer.2006;55:13-20)

(Graf et al, 2005) (Graf BA, Milbury PE, Blumberg JB. Flavonols, flavonones, flavanones and human health: Epidemological evidence. J Med Food. 2005;8:281–290)

(Guenther et al, 2006) (Guenther PM, Dodd KW, Reedy J, Krebs-Smith SM. Most Americans eat much less than recommended amounts of fruits and vegetables. J Am Diet Assoc. 2006;106:1371–1379)

(Hadi et al, 2007) (Hadi SM, Bhat SH,Azmi AS, et al.: Oxidative breakage of cellular DNA by plant polyphenols: a putative mechanism for anticancer properties. Semin Cancer Biol. 2007; 17(5): 370–376)

(Hager et al, 2008) (Hager TJ, Howard LR, Liyanage R, Lay JO, Prior RL. Ellagitannin composition of blackberry as determined by HPLC-ESI-MS and MALDI-TOF-MS. J Agric Food Chem. 2008;56(3):661–669)

(Halliwell, 1994) (Halliwell B. Free radicals, antioxidants, and human disease: curiosity, cause, or consequence? Lancet. 1994;344(8924):721–724)

(Halliwell et al, 2005) (Barry Halliwell, Joseph Rafter, and Andrew Jenner. Health promotion by flavonoids, tocopherols, tocotrienols, and other phenols: direct or indirect effects? Antioxidant or not? Am J Clin Nutr January 2005vol. 81 no. 1 268S-276S)

(Halliwell, 2007) (Halliwell B. Dietary polyphenols: Good, bad, or indifferent for your health? Cardiovasc Res. 2007;73:341–347)

(Halliwell, Gutteridge, 1989) (Halliwell, B. and Gutteridge, J.M.C. Free Radicals in Biology and Medicine, 2nd edn. Clarendon Press, Oxford, 1989)

(Hannum, 2004) (Hannum SM. Potential impact of strawberries on human health: a review of the science. Crit Rev Food Sci Nutr. 2004;44(1):1–17)

(Hartmann et al, 2008) (Hartmann A, Patz CD, Andlauer W, Dietrich H. Ludwig M. Influence of processing on quality parameters of strawberries. J Agric Food Chem. 2008;56:9484–9489)

(Harwood et al, 2007) (Harwood et al, A critical review of the data related to safety of quercetin and lack of evidence of in vivo toxicity, including lack of genotoxic/carcinogenic properties. Food and Chemical Toxicology 45, 2179-2205)

(Haseen et al, 2009) (Haseen F, Cantwell MM, O'Sullivan JM, Murray LJ. Is there a benefit from lycopene supplementation in men with prostate cancer? A systematic review. Prostate Cancer Prostatic Dis. 2009;12(4):325-32)

(Hasse et al, 2003) (Haase I, Evans R, Pofahl R, Watt FM. Regulation of keratinocyte shape, migration and wound epithelialization by igf-1- and egf-dependent signalling pathways. Journal of Cell Science. 2003;116(Pt 15):3227–3238)

(Hayes et al, 1999) (Hayes RB, Ziegler RG, Gridley G, Swanson C, Greenberg RS, Swanson GM, Schoenberg JB, Silverman DT, Brown LM, Pottern LM, Liff J, Schwartz AG, Fraumeni JF, Jr, Hoover RN. Cancer Epidemiol Biomarkers Prev. 1999;8:25–34)

(Hect et al, 1999) (Hecht, S.S., Kenney, P.M., Wang, M., Trushin, H.N., Agarwal, S., Rao, A.V. and Upadhyaya, P. (1999) Evaluation of butylated hydroxyanisole, myo-inositol, curcumin, esculetin, resveratrol and lycopene as inhibitors of benzo[a]pyrene plus

4-(methylnitrosamino)-1-(3-pyridyl)-1-butanone-induced lung tumorigenesis in A/J mice. Cancer Lett., 137, 123–130)

(Heinonen et al, 1998) (Heinonen IM, Meyer AS, Frankel EN. Antioxidant activity of berry phenolics on human low-density lipoprotein and liposome oxidation. J Agric Food Chem. 1998;46(10):4107–4112)

(Hennekens et al, 1996) (Hennekens CH, Buring JE, Manson JE, Stampfer M, Rosner B, Cook NR, Belanger C, L aMotte F, Gaziano JM, Ridker PM, et al. Lack of effect of long-term supplementation with beta carotene on the incidence of malignant neoplasms and cardiovascular disease. N Engl J Med 1996;334:1145–9)

(Hertog et al, 1995) (Hertog MG, Kromhout D, Aravanais C et al. Flavonoid intake and long-term risk of coronary heart disease and cancer in the seven countries study. Arch Intern Med 1995; 155: 381-6)

(Hertog et al, 1997) (Hertog MG, Sweetnam PM, Fehily AM, Elwood PC, Kromhout D. Antioxidant flavonols and ischemic heart disease in a Welsh population of men: the Caerphilly Study. Am J Clin Nutr 1997; 65: 1489-94)

(Hirvonen et al, 2001) (Hirvonen T, Pietinen P, Virtanen M et al. Intake of flavonols and flavones and risk of coronary heart disease in male smokers. Epidemiology 2001; 12: 62-7)

(Hollman et al, 1997) (Hollman PC, Tijburg LB, Yang CS. Bioavailability of flavonoids from tea. Crit Rev Food Sci Nutr. 1997;37:719–738)

(Holzapfel et al, 2013) (Holzapfel NP, Holzapfel BM, Champ S, Feldthusen J, Clements J, Hutmacher DW. The potential role of lycopene for the prevention and therapy of prostate cancer: from molecular mechanisms to clinical evidence. Int J Mol Sci. 2013 Jul 12;14(7):14620-46. doi: 10.3390/ijms140714620)

(Huang et al, 2012) (Wu-yang Huang, Hong-cheng Zhang, Wen-xu Liu, and Chun-yang Li. Survey of antioxidant capacity and phenolic composition of blueberry, blackberry, and strawberry in Nanjing J Zhejiang Univ Sci B. Feb 2012; 13(2): 94–102)

(Human Effect Matrix For Blueberries, 2013) (http://examine.com/supplements/Blueberry/)

(Hurst et al, 2008) (Hurst WJ, Glinski JA, Miller KB, Apgar J, Davey MH, Stuart DA (September 2008). "Survey of the trans-resveratrol and trans-piceid content of cocoa-containing and chocolate products". Journal of Agricultural and Food Chemistry 56 (18): 8374–8)

(Hurst et al, 2010) (Hurst RD, Wells RW, Hurst SM, McGhie TK, Cooney JM, Jensen DW: Blueberry fruit polyphenolics suppress oxidative stress induced skeletal muscle cell damage in vitro. Mol Nutr Food Res 2010, 54(3):353-363)

(Hwang et al, 2004) (Hwang ES, Bowen PE. Cell cycle arrest and induction of apoptosis by lycopene in Incap human prostate cancer cells. Journal of Medicinal Food. 2004;7(3):284–289)

(Imaida et al, 2001) (Imaida K, Tamano S, Kato K, Ikeda Y, Asamoto M, Takahashi S, et al. Lack of chemopreventive effects of lycopene and curcumin on experimental rat prostate carcinogenesis. Carcinogenesis.2001;22(3):467–472)

(Iqbal et al, 2008) (Iqbal R, Anand S, Ounpuu S, et al. INTERHEART Study Investigators. Dietary patterns and the risk of acute myocardial infarction in 52 countries: results of the INTERHEART study. Circulation.2008;118:1929–1937)

(Ivanov et al, 2007) (Ivanov NI, Cowell SP, Brown P, Rennie PS, Guns ES, Cox ME. Lycopene differentially induces quiescence and apoptosis in androgen-responsive and -independent prostate cancer cell lines. Clinical Nutrition. 2007;26(2):252–263)

(Jacobi, 2008) (Jacobi D. The savory side of chocolate. American Institute for Cancer Research website. Available at http://www.aicr.org/site/News2?abbr=pr_hf_&page=NewsArticle&id=9161. Accessed Jul 2014)

(Janszky et al, 2009) (Janszky I, Mukamal KJ, Ljung R, Ahnve S, Ahlbom A, Hallqvist J. Chocolate consumption and mortality following a first acute myocardial infarction: the Stockholm Heart Epidemiology Program. J Intern Med 266:248–257, 2009)

(Jatoi et al, 2007) (Jatoi A, Burch P, Hillman D, et al. A tomato-based, lycopene-containing intervention for androgen-independent prostate cancer: results of a Phase II study from the North Central Cancer Treatment Group. Urology. 2007;69:289-294)

(Jian et al, 2005) (Jian L, Du CJ, Lee AH, Binns CW. Int J Cancer. 2005;113:1010–1014)

(Jin et al, 2012) (Jin H, Leng Q, Li C. Dietary flavonoid for preventing colorectal neoplasms. Cochrane Database Syst Rev. 2012 Aug 15;8: CD009350)

(Jinyao et al, 2013) (Jinyao Chen, Yang Song, and Lishi Zhang. Effect of Lycopene Supplementation on Oxidative Stress: An Exploratory Systematic Review and Meta-Analysis of Randomized Controlled Trials. J Med Food. May 2013; 16(5): 361–374)

(Johanningsmeier, Harris, 2011) (Johanningsmeier, S.D. and Harris, G.K. Pomegranate as a Functional Food and Nutraceutical Source. Suzanne D. Johanningsmeier and G. Keith Harris. Annu Rev Food Sci Technol. 2011; 2: 181-201)

(Kalt et al, 2008) (Kalt W, Foote K, Fillmore SAE, Lyon M, van Lunen TA, McRae KB. Effect of blueberry feeding on plasma lipids in pigs. Br J Nutr. 2008;100(1):70–78)

(Kanti, Rizvi, 2009) (Kanti Bhooshan Pandey and Syed Ibrahim Rizvi. Plant polyphenols as dietary antioxidants in human health and disease. Oxid Med Cell Longev. 2009 Nov-Dec; 2(5): 270–278)

(Kaplan et al, 1990) (Kaplan LA, Lau JM, Stein EA. Clin Physiol Biochem. 1990;8:1–10)

(Kasagi et al, 2006) (Kasagi S, Seyama K, Mori H, Souma S, Sato T, Akiyoshi T, Suganuma H, Fukuchi Y. Am J Physiol Lung Cell Mol Physiol. 2006;290: L396–L404)

(Kavanaugh et al, 2007) (Kavanaugh CJ, Trumbo PR, Ellwood KC. The U.S. Food and Drug Administration's evidence-based review for qualified health claims: tomatoes, lycopene, and cancer. Journal of the National Cancer Institute. 2007;99:1074-85)

(Kavitha et al, 2013) (Kavitha K, et al. Chemopreventive effects of diverse dietary phytochemicals against DMBA-induced hamster buccal pouch carcinogenesis via the induction of Nrf2-mediated cytoprotective antioxidant, detoxification, and DNA repair enzymes. Biochimie. (2013)

(Kay, Holub, 2002) (Kay CD, Holub BJ. The effect of wild blueberry (Vaccinium angustifolium) consumption on postprandial serum antioxidant status in human subjects. Br J Nutr. (2002)

(Key et al, 2007) (Key TJ, Appleby PN, Allen NE, Travis RC, Roddam AW, Jenab M, Egevad L, Tjonneland A, Johnsen NF, Overvad K, Linseisen J, Rohrmann S, Boeing H, Pischon T, Psaltopoulou T, Trichopoulou A, Trichopoulos D, Palli D, Vineis P, Tumino R, Berrino F, Kiemeney L, Bueno-de-Mesquita HB, Quiros JR, Gonzalez CA, Martinez C, Larranaga N, Chirlaque MD, Ardanaz E, Stattin P, Hallmans G, Khaw KT, Bingham S, Slimani N, Ferrari P, Rinaldi S, Riboli E. Am J Clin Nutr. 2007;86:672–681)

(Kiani et al, 2007) (Kiani J, Imam S. Medicinal importance of grapefruit juice and its interaction with various drugs. Nutr J. 2007;6:33)

(Kim et al, 1997) (Kim, D.J., Takasuka, N., M., K.J., Sekine, K., Ota, T., Asamoto, M., Murakoshi, M., Nishino, H., Nir, Z. and Tsuda, H. (1997) Chemoprevention by lycopene of mouse lung neoplasia after combined initiation treatment with DEN, MNU and DMH. Cancer Lett., 120, 15–22)

(Kim et al, 2013) (Kim JY, et al. Oxidation of fatty acid may be enhanced by a combination of pomegranate fruit phytochemicals and acetic acid in HepG2 cells. Nutr Res Pract. (2013)

(Kirkorian et al, 2010) (Krikorian R, et al. Blueberry supplementation improves memory in older adults. J Agric Food Chem. (2010)

(Kirsh et al, 2006) (Kirsh VA, Mayne ST, Peters U, Chatterjee N, Leitzmann MF, Dixon LB, Urban DA, Crawford ED, Hayes RB. Cancer Epidemiol Biomarkers Prev. 2006;15:92–9)

(Kirsh, Mayne et al, 2006) (Kirsh VA, Mayne ST, Peters U, et al. A prospective study of lycopene and tomato product intake and risk of prostate cancer. Cancer Epidemiology, Biomarkers & Prevention. 2006;15:92-98)

(Ko, Sabanegh, 2014) (Ko EY, Sabanegh ES. The role of nutraceuticals in male fertility. Urol Clin North Am. 2014;41:181–93)

(Krasovskaya, 2012) (Valeriya Krasovskaya. Thesis: Antioxidant Properties of Berries: Review of Human Studies and their Relevance in the Context of the European Food Safety Authority. June 2012. Hogeschool van Amsterdam. http://kennisbank.hva.nl/document/478688)

(Krikorian et al, 2010, BJNutr) (Krikorian R, et al. Concord grape juice supplementation improves memory function in older adults with mild cognitive impairment. Br J Nutr. (2010)

(Krikorian et al, 2010) (Krikorian R, Shidler MD, Nash TA, Kalt W, Vinqvist-Tymchuk MR, Shukitt-Hale B, Joseph JA. Blueberry supplementation improves memory in older adults. J Agric Food Chem. 2010;58(7):3996–4000)

(Krishnamoorthy et al, 2013) (Krishnamoorthy G, Selvakumar K, Venkataraman P, Elumalai P, Arunakaran J. Lycopene supplementation prevents reactive oxygen species mediated apoptosis in Sertoli cells of adult albino rats exposed to polychlorinated biphenyls. Interdiscip Toxicol. 2013 Jun;6(2):83-92. doi: 10.2478/intox-2013-0015)

(Kroon et al, 2004) (Kroon P, Clifford M, Crozier A, et al. How should we assess the effects of exposure to dietary polyphenols in vitro. Am J Clin Nutr. 2004;80:15–21)

(Kucuk et al, 2001) (Kucuk O, Sarkar FH, Sakr W, Djuric Z, Pollak MN, Khachik F, Li YW, Banerjee M, Grignon D, Bertram JS, Crissman JD, Pontes EJ, Wood DP., Jr Cancer Epidemiol Biomarkers Prev. 2001;10:861–868)

(Landbo, Almdal, 1998) (Landbo C, Almdal TP. [Interaction between warfarin and coenzyme Q10]. [Article in Danish] Ugeskr Laeger 1998;160(22):3226-7)

(Lawenda et al, 2008) (Lawenda BD, Kelly KM, Ladas EJ, Sagar SM, Vickers A, Blumberg JB. Should supplemental antioxidant administration be avoided during chemotherapy and radiation therapy? J Natl Cancer Inst. 2008;100:773-783)

(Layher et al, 2013) (Layher JW Jr, Poling JS, Ishihara M, Azadi P, Alvarez-Manilla G, Puett D. A Possible Effect of Concentrated Oolong Tea Causing Transient Ischemic Attack-Like Symptoms. Br J Med Med Res. 2013 Jul 18;3(4):2157-2172)

(Le Marchand et al, 1991) (Le Marchand L, Hankin JH, Kolonel LN, Wilkens LR. Am J Epidemiol. 1991;133:215–219)

(Lesser et al, 2013) (A randomized, double-blind, placebo-controlled study of oral coenzyme Q10 to relieve self-reported treatment-related fatigue in newly diagnosed patients with breast cancer. Lesser GJ, Case D, Stark N, Williford S, Giguere J, Garino LA, Naughton MJ, Vitolins MZ, Lively MO, Shaw EG; J Support Oncol. 2013 Mar;11(1):31-42) a randomized, double-blind, placebo-controlled study)

(Lindshield, Erdman, 2006) (Lindshield BL, Erdman JW. In: Present Knowledge in Nutrition. Bowman BA, Russell RM, editors. Washington, D.C: International Life Sciences Institute; 2006. pp. 184–197)

(Liu et al, 2002) (Liu M, Li XQ, Weber C, Lee CY, Brown J, Liu RH. Antioxidant and antiproliferative activities of raspberries. J Agric Food Chem. 2002;50(10):2926–2930) (Ratnam et al, 2006) (Ratnam VD, Ankola DD, Bhardwaj V, Sahana DK, Kumar RMNV. Role of antioxidants in prophylaxis and therapy: a pharmaceutical perspective. J Control Release. 2006;113(3):189–207)

(Liu et al, 2013) (Liu W, et al. Cytosolic protection against ultraviolet induced DNA damage by blueberry anthocyanins and anthocyanidins in hepatocarcinoma HepG2 cells. Biotechnol Lett. (2013)

(Lohachoompol et al, 2004) (Lohachoompol, V., Srzednicki, G., Craske, J. The Change of Total Anthocyanins in Blueberries and Their Antioxidant Effect After Drying and Freezing. Journal of Biomedicine and Biotechnology (2004). 2004 (5):
248–252)

(Lu et al, 2001) (Lu QY, Hung JC, Heber D, Go VL, Reuter VE, Cordon-Cardo C, et al. Inverse associations between plasma lycopene and other carotenoids and prostate cancer. Cancer Epidemiology, Biomarkers & Prevention. 2001;10(7):749–756)

(MacDonald et al, 2009) (MacDonald L, Foster BC, Akhtar H. Food and therapeutic product interactions—A therapeutic perspective. Journal of Pharmacy & Pharmaceutical Sciences. 2009;12(3):367–377)

(Madmani et al, 2014) (Madmani ME, Yusuf Solaiman A, Tamr Agha K, Madmani Y, Shahrour Y, Essali A, Kadro W. Coenzyme Q10 for heart failure. Cochrane Database Syst Rev. 2014 Jun 2;6: CD008684. doi: 10.1002/14651858.CD008684.pub2)

(Magbanua et al, 2011) (Magbanua MJ, Roy R, Sosa EV, Weinberg V, Federman S, Mattie MD, Hughes-Fulford M, Simko J, Shinohara K, Haqq CM, Carroll PR, Chan JM. Gene expression and biological pathways in tissue of men with prostate cancer in a randomized clinical trial of lycopene and fish oil supplementation. PLoS One. 2011;6(9): e24004. doi: 10.1371/journal.pone.0024004. Epub 2011 Sep 1)

(Martin, Appel, 2010) (Martin KR, Appel CL. Polyphenols as dietary supplements: A double-edged sword. Nutrition and Dietary Supplements 2010:2)

Prof Randolph M Howes MD,PhD

(Mayo Clinic. org) (http://www.mayoclinic.org/drugs-supplements/co-enzyme-q10/evidence/hrb-20059019 (Accessed 12-23-14)

(Mayne et al, 1999) (Mayne ST, Cartmel B, Silva F, Kim CS, Fallon BG, Briskin K, Zheng T, Baum M, Shor-Posner G, Goodwin WJ., Jr J Nutr. 1999;129:849–854)

(McAnulty et al, 2004) (McAnulty SR, McAnulty LS, Nieman DC, Dumke CL, Morrow JD, Utter AC, Henson DA, Proulx WR, George GL: Consumption of blueberry polyphenols reduces exercise-induced oxidative stress compared to vitamin C. Nutrition Res 2004, 24(3):209-221)

(McAnulty et la, 2005) (McAnulty SR, McAnulty LS, Morrow JD, Khardouni D, Shooter L, Monk J, Gross S, Brown V: Effect of daily fruit ingestion on angiotensin converting enzyme activity, blood pressure, and oxidative stress in chronic smokers. Free Rad Res 2005, 39(11):1241-1248)

(McAnulty et al, 2011) (McAnulty LS, et al. Effect of blueberry ingestion on natural killer cell counts, oxidative stress, and inflammation prior to and after 2.5 h of running. Appl Physiol Nutr Metab. (2011)

(McCann et al, 2005) (McCann SE, Ambrosone CB, Moysich KB, Brasure J, Marshall JR, Freudenheim JL, Wilkinson GS, Graham S. Nutr Cancer. 2005;53:33–41)

(McGinley, Shafat, 2009) (McGinley C, Shafat A: Does antioxidant vitamin supplementation protect against muscle damage? Sports Med 2009, 39(12):1011-1032)

(McLeay et al, 2012) (McLeay Y, et al. Effect of New Zealand blueberry consumption on recovery from eccentric exercise-induced muscle damage. J Int Soc Sports Nutr. (2012)

(Med Ltr, 2006) (Coenzyme Q10 (2006). Medical Letter on Drugs and Therapeutics, 48(1229): 19–20)

(Mendiola et al, 2010) (Mendiola J, Torres-Cantero AM, Vioque J, Moreno-Grau JM, Ten J, et al. A low intake of antioxidant nutrients is associated with poor semen quality in patients attending fertility clinics. Fertil Steril. 2010;93:1128–33)

(Miller et al, 2002) (Miller EC, Hadley CW, Schwartz SJ, Erdman JW, Jr, Boileau TW-M, Clinton SK. Lycopene, tomato products, and prostate cancer prevention. Have we established causality? Pure and Applied Chemistry. 2002;74(8):1435–1441)

(Mink et al, 2007) (Mink PJ, Scrafford CG, Barraj LM, et al. Flavonoid intake and cardiovascular disease mortality: a prospective study in post-menopausal women. Am J Clin Nutr. 2007;85:895–909)

(Moghe et al, 2012) (Moghe SS, et al. Effect of blueberry polyphenols on 3T3-F442A preadipocyte differentiation. J Med Food. (2012)

(Moran et al, 2013) (Nancy E. Moran, John W. Erdman, Jr., and Steven K. Clinton. Complex interactions between dietary and genetic factors impact lycopene metabolism and distribution. Arch Biochem Biophys. Nov 15, 2013; 539(2): 10.1016/j.abb.2013.06.017)

(Morre, Morre, 2005) (Morre DM, Morre DJ. Anticancer activity of grape and grape skin extracts alone and combined with green tea infusions. Cancer Lett 2005; 26: (Epub ahead of print)

(Mossine et al, 2008) (Mossine VV, Chopra P, Mawhinney TP. Interaction of tomato lycopene and ketosamine against rat prostate tumorigenesis. Cancer Research. 2008;68(11):4384–4391)

(Mursu et al, 2004) (Mursu, J., Voutilainen, S., Nurmi, T., Rissanen, T., Virtanen, J., & Kaikkonen, J.,...Salonen, J. (2004). "Dark chocolate consumption increases HDL cholesterol concentration and chocolate fatty acids may inhibit lipid peroxidation in healthy humans". Free Radical Biology & Medicine 37 (9): 1351–1359)

(Murtaugh et al, 2004) (Murtaugh MA, Ma KN, Benson J, Curtin K, Caan B, Slattery ML. Am J Epidemiol. 2004;159:32–41)

(Myung et al, 2013) (Myung SK, Ju W, Cho B, Oh SW, Park SM, Koo BK, Park BJ; Korean Meta-Analysis Study Group. Efficacy of vitamin and antioxidant supplements in prevention of cardiovascular disease: systematic review and meta-analysis of randomised controlled trials. BMJ. 2013 Jan 18;346: f10. doi: 10.1136/bmj.f10)

(Nagasawa et al, 1995) (Nagasawa, H., Mitamura, T., Sakamoto, S. and Yamamoto, K. (1995) Effects of lycopene on spontaneous mammary tumour development in SHN virgin mice. Anticancer Res., 15, 1173–1178)

(Nardini et al, 2007) (Nardini M, Natella F, Scaccini C. Role of dietary polyphenols in platelet aggregation. A review of the supplementation studies. Platelets. 2007;18:224–243)

(NCI, 2010) (National Cancer Institute. Promises and perils of lycopene/tomato supplementation and cancer prevention. (Executive summary

of February 17-18, 2005 conference) Accessed at http://dcp.cancer.gov/
Files/news-events/20050217-18e.pdf on March 4, 2010)

(NCI, 2012) (National Cancer Institute (2012). Coenzyme Q10 (PDQ)
– Health Professional Version. Available online: http://cancer.gov/can-
certopics/pdq/cam/coenzymeQ10/healthprofessional)   (Accessed
12-23-14)

(NET-PD, 2007) (A randomized clinical trial of coenzyme Q10
and GPI-1485 in early Parkinson disease. Neurology. 2007 Jan
2;68(1):20-8)

(Netzel et al, 2002) (Netzel M, Strass G, Kaul C, et al. In vivo antioxidative capacity of a composite berry juice. Food Res Int.
2002;35:213–216)

(Neuman et al, 2000) (Neuman I, Nahum H, Ben-Amotz A. Reduction of
exercise-induced asthma oxidative stress by lycopene, a natural antioxidant. Allergy. 2000;55:1184-1189)

(Nieman et al, 2004) (Nieman DC, Henson DA, McAnulty SR, McAnulty
LS, Morrow JD, Ahmed A, Heward CB: Vitamin E and immunity after
the Kona Triathlon World Championship. Med Sci Sports Exerc 2004,
36:1328-1335)

(Nieman, Stear, 2010) (Nieman DC, Stear S: A–Z of nutritional supplements: dietary supplements, sports nutrition foods and ergogen-
ic aids for health and performance: part 15. Br J Sports Med 2010,
44(16):1202-1206)

(Norrish et al,2000) (NorrishAE,Jackson RT,Sharpe SJ,Skeaff CM.Prostate
cancer and dietary carotenoids. Am J Epidemiol.2000;151:119-123)

(Obermuller-Jevic et al, 2003) (Obermuller-Jevic UC, Olano-Martin E,
Corbacho AM, Eiserich JP, van der Vliet A, Valacchi G, et al. Lycopene in-
hibits the growth of normal human prostate epithelial cells in vitro. The
Journal of Nutrition. 2003;133(11):3356–3360)

(Okajima et al, 1997) (Okajima, E., Ozono, S., Endo, T., Majima, T.,
Tsutsumi, M., Fukuda, T., Akai, H., Denda, A., Hirao, Y., Nishino, H., Nir,
Z. and Konishi, Y. (1997) Chemopreventive efficacy of piroxicam administered alone or in combination with lycopene and beta-carotene
on the development of rat urinary bladder carcinoma after N-butyl-
N-(4-hydroxybutyl)nitrosamine treatment. Jpn. J. Cancer Res., 88,
543–552)

(Olesen et al, 2014) (Olesen J, Gliemann L, Biensø R, Schmidt J, Hellsten Y, Pilegaard H. Exercise training, but not resveratrol, improves metabolic and inflammatory status in skeletal muscle of aged men. J Physiol. 2014 Apr 15;592(Pt 8):1873-86)

(Oransky, 2012) (Oransky I. Retraction count for resveratrol researcher Dipak Das rises to 12. Retraction Watch Web site, June 3, 2012)

(Paiva, Russell, 1999) (Paiva SA, Russell RM. Beta-carotene and other carotenoids as antioxidants. J Am Coll Nutr. 1999;18:426-433)

(Pakrashi, Oihninger, 2014) (Tarita Pakrashi and Sergio Oehninger. Lycopene and male infertility: do we know enough? Asian J Androl. 2014 May-Jun; 16(3): 500)

(Peters et al, 2001) (Peters U, Poole C, Arab L. Does tea affect cardiovascular disease? A meta-analysis. Am J Epidemiol. 2001;154:495–503)

(Peralta, Spooner, 2007) (Peralta IE, Spooner DM. History, origin and early cultivation of tomato (Solanaceae) In: Razdan MK, Mattoo AK, editors. Genetic improvement of solanaceous crops. Vol. 2. 2007. pp. 1–27)

(Peters et al, 2007) (Peters U, Leitzmann MF, Chatterjee N, Wang Y, Albanes D, Gelmann EP, Friesen MD, Riboli E, Hayes RB. Cancer Epidemiol Biomarkers Prev. 2007;16:962–968)

(Peters, Leitzmann et al, 2007) (Peters U, Leitzmann MF, Chatterjee N, et al. Serum Lycopene, Other Carotenoids, and Prostate Cancer Risk: a Nested Case-Control Study in the Prostate, Lung, Colorectal, and Ovarian Cancer Screening Trial. Cancer Epidemiol Biomarkers Prev. 2007 16: 962-968)

(Petr, Erdman, 2005) (Petr L, Erdman JW. Lycopne and risk of cardiovascular disease. In: Packer L, Obermuller-Jevic U, Kraemer K, Sies H, editors. Carotenoids and Retinoids: Molecular Aspects and Health Issues. Champaign: AOCS Press; 2005. pp. 204–217)

(Pourmand et al, 2007) (Pourmand G, Salem S, Mehrsai A, Lotfi M, Amirzargar MA, Mazdak H, Roshani A, Kheirollahi A, Kalantar E, Baradaran N, Saboury B, Allameh F, Karami A, Ahmadi H, Jahani Y. Asian Pac J Cancer Prev. 2007;8:422–428)

(Prior et al, 2007) (Prior R.L., Gu L., Wu X., Jacob R.A., Sotoudeh G., Kader A.A., Cook R.A. Plasma Antioxidant Capacity Changes Following a Meal as a Measure of the Ability of a Food to Alter In Vivo Antioxidant

Prof Randolph M Howes MD,PhD

Status. Journal of the American College of Nutrition (2007). 26 (2): 170–181)

(Prior et al, 2009) (Prior RL, Wu X, Gu L, et al. Purified berry anthocyanins but not whole berries normalize lipid parameters in mice fed an obesogenic high fat diet. Mol Nutr Food Res. 2009;53:1406–1418)

(Raitakari et al, 2000) (Raitakari OT, McCredie RJ, Witting P, Griffiths KA, Letters J, Sullivan D, Stocker R, Celermajer DS. Coenzyme Q improves LDL resistance to ex vivo oxidation but does not enhance endothelial function in hypercholesterolemic young adults. Free Radic Biol Med. 2000 Apr 1;28(7):1100-5)

(Raj et al, 2014) (Raj MV, Selvakumar K, Krishnamoorthy G, Revathy S, Elumalai P, et al. Impact of lycopene on epididymal androgen and estrogen receptors' expression in polychlorinated biphenyls-exposed rat. Reprod Sci. 2014;21:89–101)

(Rao, Agarwal, 1998) (Rao AV, Agarwal S. Bioavailability and in vivo antioxidant properties of lycopene from tomato products and their possible role in the prevention of cancer. Nutr Cancer. 1998;31:199-203)

(Reid et al, 2010) (Ried K, Sullivan T, Fakler P, Frank OR, Stocks NP. Does chocolate reduce blood pressure? A meta-analysis. BMC Med. 2010 Jun 28;8:39)

(Renaud, de Lorgeril, 1992) (Renaud S, de Lorgeril M. Wine, alcohol, platelets, and the French paradox for coronary heart disease. Lancet. 1992;339:1523–1526)

(Rimm et al, 1996) (Rimm EB, Katan MB, Ascherio A, Stampfer MJ, Willett WC. Relation between intake of flavonoids and risk for coronary heart disease in male health professionals. Ann Intern Med 1996; 125: 384-9)

(Rizvi et al, 2005) (Rizvi SI, Zaid MA, Anis R, Mishra N. Protective role of tea catechins against oxidation-induced damage of type 2 diabetic erythrocytes. Clin Exp Pharmacol Physiol. 2005;32:70–75)

(Rizvi, Zaid, 2001) (Rizvi S I, Zaid M A. Insulin like effect of epicatechin on membrane acetylcholinesterase activity in type 2 diabetes mellitus. Clin Exp Pharmacol Physiol. 2001;28:776–778)

(Rodrigo et al, 2013) (Rodrigo R, Libuy M, Feliú F, Hasson D. Molecular basis of cardioprotective effect of antioxidant vitamins in myocardial infarction. Biomed Res Int. 2013;2013:437613. doi: 10.1155/2013/437613. Epub 2013 Jul 14)

(Rolfes, Whitney, 2009) (Rolfes S.R., Pinna K. and Whitney E. Understanding normal and clinical nutrition. 8th edition. Wadsworth Cengage Learning, 2009)

(Rosenblat et al, 2006) (Rosenblat, M., Hayek, T., Aviram, M. Anti-oxidative effects of pomegranate juice (PJ) consumption by diabetic patients on serum and on macrophages. Atherosclerosis. 2006. Aug. 187: 363–71)

(Ross, 2009) (Ross, S.M. Pomegranate. Its Role in Cardiovascular Health. Stephanie Maxine Ross. Holist Nurs Pract, 2009; 23(3): 195–197)

(Ross et al, 2010) (Ross C, Morriss A, Khairy M, Khalaf Y, Braude P, et al. A systematic review of the effect of oral antioxidants on male infertility. Reprod Biomed Online. 2010;20:711–23)

(Ruel et al, 2008) (Ruel G, Pomerleau S, Couture P, Lemieux S, Lamarche B, Couillard C. Low-calorie cranberry juice supplementation reduces plasma oxidized LDL and cell adhesion molecule concentrations in men. Br J Nutr. 2008;99:352–359)

(Scalbert et al, 2005) (Scalbert A, Manach C, Morand C, Remesy C. Dietary polyphenols and the prevention of diseases. Crit Rev Food Sci Nutr. 2005;45:287–306)

(Sanderson et al, 2004) (Sanderson M, Coker AL, Logan P, Zheng W, Fadden MK. Cancer Causes Control. 2004;15:647–655)

(Sariburun et al, 2010) (Sariburun E, Sahin S, Demir C, Türkben C, Uylaşer V. Phenolic content and antioxidant activity of raspberry and blackberry cultivars. J Food Sci. 2010;75(4): C328–C335. doi: 10.1111/j.1750-3841)

(Scarmeas et al, 2007) (Scarmeas N, Luchsinger J A, Mayeux R, Stern Y. Mediterranean diet and Alzheimer disease mortality. Neurology. 2007;69:1084–1093)

(Schilter et al, 2003) (Schilter B, Andersson C, Anton R, et al. Guidance for the safety assessment of botanicals and botanical preparations for use in food and food supplements. Food Chem Toxicol. 2003;41:1625–1649)

(Schmitz et al, 1991) (Schmitz HH, Poor CL, Wellman RB, Erdman JW., Jr J Nutr. 1991;121:1613–1621) (Kaplan et al, 1990) (Kaplan LA, Lau JM, Stein EA. Clin Physiol Biochem. 1990;8:1–10)

(Schuman et al, 1982) (Schuman LM, Mandel JS, Radke A, Seal U, Halberg F. Trends in cancer incidence: causes and practical implications. 1982:345–354)

(Scheid et al, 2010) (Scheid L, Reusch A, Stehle P, Ellinger S. Antioxidant effects of cocoa and cocoa products ex vivo and in vivo: is there evidence from controlled intervention studies? Curr Opin Clin Nutr Metab Care. 2010 Nov;13(6):737-42)

(Sekizawa et al, 2013) (Sekizawa H, et al. Relationship between polyphenol content and anti-influenza viral effects of berries. J Sci Food Agric. (2013)

(Semba et al, 2014) (Semba R et al, Resveratrol levels and all-cause mortality in older community-dwelling adults. JAMA Intern Med. 2014;174(7):1077-1084)

(Sesso, 2006) (Sesso HD. Carotenoids and cardiovascular disease: what research gaps remain? Curr Opin Lipidol. 2006 Feb;17(1):11-6)

(Sesso et al, 2007) (Sesso HD, Gaziano JM, Jenkins DJ, Buring JE. Strawberry intake, lipids, C-reactive protein, and the risk of cardiovascular disease in women. J Am Coll Nutr. 2007;26:303–310)

(Setchell et al, 2003) (Setchell KD, Faughnan MS, Avades T, Zimmer-Nechemias L, Brown NM, et al. Comparing the pharmacokinetics of daidzein and genistein with the use of 13C-labeled tracers in premenopausal women. Am J Clin Nutr. 2003;77:411–419)

(Sharp et al, 2014) (Sharp J, Farha S, Park MM, Comhair SA, Lundgrin EL, Tang WH, Bongard RD, Merker MP, Erzurum SC. Coenzyme Q supplementation in pulmonary arterial hypertension. Redox Biol. 2014 Jul 31;2:884-91. doi: 10.1016/j.redox.2014.06.010. eCollection 2014)

(Sharoni et al, 2002) (Sharoni Y, Danilenko M, Walfisch S, Amir H, Nahum A, Ben-Dor A, et al. Role of gene regulation in the anticancer activity of carotenoids. Pure and Applied Chemistry. 2002;74(8):1469–1477)

(Shaughnessy et al, 2009) (Shaughnessy KS, Boswall IA, Scanlan AP, Gottschall-Pass KT, Sweeney MI. Diets containing blueberry extract lower blood pressure in spontaneously hypertensive stroke-prone rats. Nutr Res.2009;29(2):130–138)

(Shi, Le Maguer, 2000) (Shi J, Le Maguer M. Lycopene in tomatoes: Chemical and physical properties affected by food processing. Critical Reviews in Biotechnology. 2000;20(4):293–334)

(Shukitt-Hale et al, 2008) (Shukitt-Hale B, et al. Blueberry polyphenols attenuate kainic acid-induced decrements in cognition and alter inflammatory gene expression in rat hippocampus. Nutr Neurosci. (2008)

(Shults et al, 2002) (Shults CW, Oakes D, Kieburtz K, Beal MF, Haas R, Plumb S, Juncos JL, Nutt J, Shoulson I, Carter J, Kompoliti K, Perlmutter JS, Reich S, Stern M, Watts RL, Kurlan R, Molho E, Harrison M, Lew M, . Effects of coenzyme Q10 in early Parkinson disease: evidence of slowing of the functional decline. Arch Neurol. 2002 Oct;59(10):1541-50)

(Sibai, 1998) (Sibai BM. Prevention of preeclampsia: a big disappointment. Am J Obstet Gynecol. 1998;179:1275-1278)

(Sies, Stahl, 1998) (Sies H, Stahl W. Lycopene: antioxidant and biological effects and its bioavailability in the human. Proc Soc Exp Biol Med. 1998;218:121-124)

(Sies et al, 2007) (Sies H. J Nutr. 2007;137:1493–1495)

(Sies, Stahl, Sevanian, 2005) (Sies H, Stahl W, Sevanian A. J Nutr. 2005;135:969–972)

(Slater et al, 2011) (A randomized, double-blinded, placebo-controlled, crossover, add-on study of CoEnzyme Q10 in the prevention of pediatric and adolescent migraine. Slater SK, Nelson TD, Kabbouche MA, LeCates SL, Horn P, Segers A, Manning P, Powers SW, Hershey AD. Cephalalgia. 2011 Jun;31(8):897-905)

(Smith et al, 2001) (Smith AF, Peralta IE, Spooner DM. Early history, culture, and cookery. Vol. 5. University of Illinois Press; 2001)

(Snow et al, 2010) (Snow BJ, Rolfe FL, Lockhart MM, Frampton CM, O'Sullivan JD, Fung V, Smith RA, Murphy MP, Taylor KM, . A double-blind, placebo-controlled study to assess the mitochondria-targeted antioxidant MitoQ as a disease-modifying therapy in Parkinson's disease. Mov Disord. 2010 Aug 15;25(11):1670-4)

(Sommer, Vyas, 2012) (Sommer A, Vyas KS. A global clinical view on vitamin A and carotenoids. Am J Clin Nutr.2012;96:1204S–6)

(Sonada et al, 2004) (Sonoda T, Nagata Y, Mori M, Miyanaga N, Takashima N, Okumura K, Goto K, Naito S, Fujimoto K, Hirao Y, Takahashi A, Tsukamoto T, Fujioka T, Akaza H. Cancer Sci. 2004;95:238–242)

(Spigset, 1994) (Spigset O. Reduced effect of warfarin caused by ubidecarenone. Lancet 1994;344(8933):1372-3)

(Spindler et al, 2009) (Spindler M, Beal MF, Henchcliffe C. Coenzyme Q10 effects in neurodegenerative disease. Neuropsychiatr Dis Treat. 2009;5:597-610)

(Srivastava et al, 2007) (Srivastava A, Akoh CC, Fischer J, Krewer G. Effect of anthocyanin fractions from selected cultivars of Georgia-grown blueberries on apoptosis and phase II enzymes. J Agric Food Chem.2007;55(8):3180–3185)

(Stauth, 2007) (Stauth, David (5 March 2007) Studies force new view on biology of flavonoids, EurekAlert!. Adapted from a news release issued by Oregon State University)

(Stull et al, 2010) (Stull AJ, et al. Bioactives in blueberries improve insulin sensitivity in obese, insulin-resistant men and women. J Nutr. (2010)

(Talvas et al, 2010) (Talvas J. Caris-Veyrat C. Guy L, et al. Differential effects of lycopene consumed in tomato paste and lycopene in the form of a purified extract on target genes of cancer prostatic cells. Am J Clin Nutr.2010;91:1716–1724)

(Tan et al, 2010) (Tan Hsueh-Li, Jennifer M. Thomas-Ahner, Elizabeth M. Grainger, Lei Wan, David M. Francis, Steven J. Schwartz, John W. Erdman, Jr., and Steven K. Clinton. Tomato-based food products for prostate cancer prevention: what have we learned? Cancer Metastasis Rev. Sep 2010; 29(3): 10.1007/s10555-010-9246-z)

(Tang et al, 2009) (Tang FY, Cho HJ, Pai MH, Chen YH. Concomitant supplementation of lycopene and eicosapentaenoic acid inhibits the proliferation of human colon cancer cells. The Journal of Nutritional Biochemistry. 2009;20(6):426–434)

(Theodorou et al, 2011) (Theodorou AA, Nikolaidis MG, Paschalis VP, Koutsias S, Panayiotou GP, Fatouros IG, Koutedakis YK, Jamurtas AZ: No effect of antioxidant supplementation on muscle performance and blood redox status adaptations to eccentric training. Am J Clin Nut 2011, 93:1373-83)

(Thies et al, 2012) (Thies F, Masson LF, Rudd A, Vaughan N, Tsang C, et al. Effect of a tomato-rich diet on markers of cardiovascular disease risk in moderately overweight, disease-free, middle-aged adults: a randomized controlled trial. Am J Clin Nutr. 2012;95:1013–22)

(Tresserra-Rimbau et al, 2014) (Tresserra-Rimbau A, Rimm EB, Medina-Remón A, Martínez-González MA, López-Sabater MC, Covas MI, Corella D, Salas-Salvadó J, Gómez-Gracia E, Lapetra J, Arós F, Fiol M, Ros E, Serra-Majem

L, Pintó X, Muñoz MA, Gea A, Ruiz-Gutiérrez V, Estruch R, Lamuela-Raventós RM; PREDIMED Study Investigators. Polyphenol intake and mortality risk: a re-analysis of the PREDIMED trial. BMC Med. 2014 May 13;12:77)

(Tulipani et al, 2008) (Tulipani S, Mezzetti B, Capocasa F, Bompadre S, Beekwilder J, de Vos CHR, Capanoglu E, Bovy A, Battino M. Antioxidants, phenolic compounds, and nutritional quality of different strawberry genotypes. J Agric Food Chem. 2008;56(3):696–704)

(Twiddy et al, 2012) (Twiddy AL, Cox ME, Wasan KM. Prostate. 2012;72:955–965)

(UConn Today, 2012) (Scientific journals notified following research misconduct investigation. UConn Today, Jan 12, 2012)

(Vaishampayan et al, 2007) (Vaishampayan U, Hussain M, Banerjee M, Seren S, Sarkar FH, Fontana J, Forman JD, Cher ML, Powell I, Pontes JE, Kucuk O. Lycopene and soy isoflavones in the treatment of prostate cancer. Nutr Cancer. 2007;59:1-7)

(van Breeman et al, 2011) (van Breemen RB, Sharifi R, Viana M, Pajkovic N, Zhu D, Yuan L, Yang Y, Bowen PE, Stacewicz-Sapuntzakis M. Cancer Prev Res (Phila) 2011;4:711–718)

(Vang et al, 2011) (Vang O and others. What is new for an old molecule? Systematic review and recommendations on the use of resveratrol. PloS One 6(6): e19881. doi:10.1371/journal.pone.0019881, 2011)

(Voutilainen et al, 2006) (Voutilainen S, Nurmi T, Mursu J, Rissanen TH. Am J Clin Nutr. 2006;83:1265–1271)

(Walle et al, 2004) (Walle T, Hsieh F, DeLegge MH, Oatis JE, Walle UK (December 2004). "High absorption but very low bioavailability of oral resveratrol in humans". Drug Metab. Dispos. 32 (12): 1377–82)

(Wang et al, 2006) (Wang L, Liu S, Manson JE, et al. The consumption of lycopene and tomato-based food products is not associated with the risk of type 2 diabetes in women. J Nutr. 2006;136:620-625)

(Wang et al, 2010) (Wang, Bo Chu, He, Rui, Li, Zhi Min. Food Technol The Stability and Antioxidant Activity of Anthocyanins from Blueberry. Biotechnol (2010). 48 (1): 42–49)

(Wang et al, 2013) (Wang Y, et al. Dietary supplementation of blueberry juice enhances hepatic expression of metallothionein and attenuates liver fibrosis in rats. PLoS One. (2013)

(Warren et al, 1992) (Warren JA, Jenkins RR, Packer L, Witt EH, Armstrong RB: Elevated muscle vitamin E does not attenuate eccentric exercise-induced muscle injury. J Appl Physiol 1992, 72:2168-2172)

(Watts, 1995) (Watts TL. Coenzyme Q10 and periodontal treatment: is there any beneficial effect? Br Dent J 1995;178(6):209-13)

(WCRF, 1997) (World Cancer Research Fund. Food, nutrition and the prevention of cancer: A global perspective. Washington, D.C.: American Institute for Cancer Research; 1997) WCRF, 2007 (World Cancer Research Fund. Food, nutrition and the prevention of cancer: A global perspective. Washington, DC: American Institute for Cancer Research; 2007)

(Wei, Giovannucci, 2012) (Wei MY, Giovannucci EL. J Oncol. 2012;2012:271063)

(Weir et al, 2012) (Weir, William; Megan, Kathleen (January 11, 2012). "Investigation Finds UConn Professor Fabricated Research - Work Focused On Resveratrol, Chemical In Red Wine". Hartford Courant) (Retraction Watch)

(Weisburger, 1998) (Weisburger JH. Evaluation of the evidence on the role of tomato products in disease prevention. Proc Soc Exp Biol Med. 1998;218:140-143)

(Williamson, Manach, 3005) (Williamson G, Manach C. II. Bioavailability and bioefficacy of polyphenols in humans. II. Review of 93 intervention studies. Am J Clin Nutr. 2005 Jan; 81(1 Suppl): 243-255)

(Wiseman et al, 2000) (Wiseman H, O'Reilly JD, Adlercreutz H, et al. Isoflavone phytoestrogens consumed in soy decrease F_2-isoprostane concentrations and increase resistance of low-density lipoprotein to oxidation in humans. Am J Clin Nutr2000;72:395-400)

(Wilms et al, 2007) (Wilms L.C., Boots A.W., de Boer V.C., Maas L.M., Pachen D.M., Gottschalk R.W., Ketelslegers H.B., Godschalk R.W., Haenen G.R., van Schooten F.J., Kleinjans J.C. Impact of multiple genetic polymorphisms on effects of a 4-week blueberry juice intervention on ex vivo induced lymphocytic DNA damage in human volunteers. Carcinogenesis (2007). 28 (8): 1800–1806)

(Wojdylo et al, 2009) (Wojdyło A, Figiel A, Oszmiański J. Effect of drying methods with the application of vacuum microwaves on the bioactive compounds, color, and antioxidant activity of strawberry fruits. J Agric Food Chem. 2009;57:1337–1343)

(Wolfe et al, 2008) (Wolfe K.L., Kang X., He X., Dong M., Zhang Q., Liu R.H. Cellular Antioxidant Activity of Common Fruits. Journal of Agricultural and Food Chemistry (2008). 56 (18): 8418–8426)

(Wu et al, 2002) (Wu, Xianli, Cao, Guohua, Prior, Ronald L. Absorption and Metabolism of Anthocyanins in Elderly Women after Consumption of Elderberry or Blueberry. The Journal Of Nutrition (2002). 132: 1865–1871)

(Wu et al, 2004) (Wu X, Beecher GR, Holden JM, Haytowitz DB, Gebhardt SE, Prior RL: Lipophilic and hydrophilic antioxidant capacities of common foods in the United States. J Agri Food Chem 2004, 52:4026-4037)

(Wu, Erdman, Schwartz et al, 2004) (Wu K, Erdman JW, Jr, Schwartz SJ, Platz EA, Leitzmann M, Clinton SK, et al. Plasma and dietary carotenoids, and the risk of prostate cancer: A nested case–control study. Cancer Epidemiology, Biomarkers & Prevention. 2004;13(2):260–269)

(Wu et al, 2010) (Wu X, et al. Dietary blueberries attenuate atherosclerosis in apolipoprotein E-deficient mice by upregulating antioxidant enzyme expression. J Nutr. (2010)

(Xu et al, 2013) (Xu J, et al. Intake of Blueberry Fermented by Lactobacillus plantarum Affects the Gut Microbiota of L-NAME Treated Rats. Evid Based Complement Alternat Med. (2013)

(Yang et al, 2001) (Yang CS, Landau JM, Huang MT, Newmark HL. Inhibition of carcinogenesis by dietary polyphenolic compounds. Ann Rev Nutr. 2001;21:381–406)

(Yang et al, 2009) (Yang L, Zhao K, Calingasan NY, Luo G, Szeto HH, Beal MF. Mitochondria targeted peptides protect against 1-methyl-4-phenyl-1,2,3,6-tetrahydropyridine neurotoxicity. Antioxid Redox Signal. 2009 Sep;11(9)

(Ye, Yuan, 2013) (Ye Y, Li J, Yuan Z. Effect of antioxidant vitamin supplementation on cardiovascular outcomes: a meta-analysis of randomized controlled trials. PLoS One. 2013;8(2): e56803. doi: 10.1371/journal.pone.0056803. Epub 2013 Feb 20)

(Yfanti et al, 2010) (Yfanti C, Akerstrom T, Nielsen S, Nielsen AR, Mounier R, Mortensen OH, Lykkesfeldt J, Rose AJ, Fischer CP, Pedersen BK: Antioxidant supplementation does not alter endurance training adaptation. Med Sci Sports Exerc 2010, 42:1388-1395)

(Young et al, 2004) (Young AJ, Phillip DM, Lowe GM. In: Carotenoids in Health and Disease. Krinsky NI, Mayne ST, Sies H, editors. New York: Marcel Dekkar; 2004. pp. 105–126)

(Yuji et al, 2013) (Yuji K, et al. Effect of dietary blueberry (Vaccinium ashei Reade) leaves on serum and hepatic lipid levels in rats. J Oleo Sci. (2013)

(Zawiasa et al, 2009) (Zawiasa, A.; Szklarek-Kubicka, M.; Fijałkowska-Morawska, J.; Nowak, D.; Rysz, J.; Mamełka, B.; Nowicki, M. (2009). "Effect of Oral Fructose Load on Serum Uric Acid and Lipids in Kidney Transplant Recipients Treated with Cyclosporine or Tacrolimus". Transplantation Proceedings 41 (1): 188–91)

(Zhang et al, 2007) (Zhang J, Dhakal I, Stone A, Ning B, Greene G, Lang NP, Kadlubar FF. Nutr Cancer. 2007;59:46–53)

(Zheng et al, 2003) (Zheng Y, et al. Effect of high-oxygen atmospheres on blueberry phenolics, anthocyanins, and antioxidant capacity. J Agric Food Chem. (2003)

(Zheng, Wang, 2010) (Zheng W., Wang S.Y. Oxygen radical absorbing capacity of phenolics in blueberries, cranberries, chokeberries, and lingon berries. Journal of Agricultural and Food Chemistry (2010). 51 (2): 502-9)